D1194445

Keeping Abreast

**breast changes
that are
not cancer**

Kerry A. McGinn, RN, BSN, MA

with the participation of the Breast Health Center
Children's Hospital of San Francisco

**Bull Publishing Company
Palo Alto, California**

Copyright 1987 Kerry Anne McGinn

ISBN 0-915950-82-0

Bull Publishing Co.
P.O. Box 208
Palo Alto, CA 94302-0208
(415) 322-2855

Cover and interior design: Michelle Taverniti
Interior illustrations: Ken Miller
Production Manager: Helen O'Donnell

Printed in the U.S.
All rights reserved
Distributed to the trade by:
Publishers Group West
5855 Beaudry Street
Emeryville, CA 94608

Library of Congress Cataloging-in-Publication Data

McGinn, Kerry Anne.
Keeping Abreast

1. Breast—Diseases—Popular works. I. Children's
Hospital of San Francisco. Breast Health Center.
II. Title. [DNLM: 1. Breast Diseases—popular
works. WP 840 M478k]
RG491.M38   1987   618.1'9   87-15855
ISBN 0-91595-82-0

The comments made by Ann Jillian are an
endorsement of *Keeping Abreast* and *not* an
endorsement of The Breast Health Center at
Children's Hospital, San Francisco, or any other
particular breast health center.

Dedicated with love to two special young women:
my daughter Kathleen and my daughter-in-law Susan

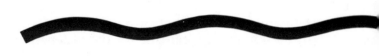

Contents

Dear Reader,

This book happened because I was worried and bewildered about changes in my own breasts. As I talked to other women, I found that many of them shared my concerns—and that few of them were getting the answers they needed.

I was fortunate enough to discover the Breast Health Center at Children's Hospital of San Francisco. They helped me, and then agreed to collaborate on a book to share their information and practical counsel with women everywhere.

This book is not about breast cancer. It's about all the breast changes that aren't breast cancer, from the most innocent general lumpiness through breast carcinoma in situ (noninvasive breast carcinoma)—a topic of special interest to the breast team at Children's Hospital. (Doctors still disagree on whether breast carcinoma in situ is properly classified as the last stage in a continuum of benign breast changes or as an early cancer.)

My thanks go to the members (current and former) of the breast health team at Children's Hospital: Cathy Coleman, R.N., nurse specialist; Patricia T. Kelly, Ph.D., medical geneticist; Michael D. Lagios, M.D., pathologist; Frederick Margolin, M.D., radiologist; Pat Kizpolski McCarthy, R.N., MSN, oncology nurse consultant; Jon Ross, M.D., pathologist; and Philip Westdahl, M.D., surgeon. Not only did they provide information and moral support, but also editorial review of the manuscript. I am also grateful to Virginia Griswold, M.D., radiologist; David A. Wood, M.D., cancer researcher; Carolyn Gale Anderson, masseuse; and Edwin Silverberg, statistician, American Cancer Society, New York for their assistance.

I thank the members of my own breast health team: Peter Sapienza, M.D., surgeon and Richard Dorsay, M.D., radiologist with the Kaiser-Permanente

Medical Center, South San Francisco; and Susan Bertolli, M.D., gynecologist, and Anne Fukutome, M.D., internist with Kaiser, San Francisco. And, as always, I'm grateful to David Bull, my capable and enthusiastic publisher.

And, finally, thank you to my husband, Art; my children, Mike, Kathy, John (and daughter-in-law Sue), and Steve; and my father, Robert Mullen, for their unceasing encouragement.

As a woman, a patient, a nurse, a mother, a daughter, and a friend (not necessarily in that order)—I thank you all.

Fondly,
Kerry Anne McGinn

Keeping
Abreast

"**M**y nurse practitioner found something in my breast yesterday. She wants me to see a doctor in two weeks."

Patrice's voice was light, her manner carefully casual as we chatted in the dressing room after our dance class—but conversations hushed suddenly. Faces turned toward Patrice.

Lillian broke the silence. "How awful. I hope it turns out okay."

"My doctor says I have fibrocystic disease in my breasts," contributed Gloriana. "It worries me—and sometimes it really hurts. No one seems to know what to do about it, and some people say it can lead to cancer."

"I've heard that giving up coffee helps," offered Elizabeth.

And Kathie, speaking very softly: "I can't make myself go to the doctor. I know I should, but the whole idea panics me. I think there might be a lump in one of my breasts. My mother had breast cancer and I'm scared."

Patrice again: "It's the waiting that gets me. I don't want to stew about it for two weeks."

This book is for...

This book is for all the Patrices and Glorianas and Kathies.

It is *not* for the woman with a new diagnosis of breast cancer. She can check her bookstore and library for numerous books about her treatment choices.

Instead, this book is for the rest of us. It's for every woman with lumpy, bumpy breasts, with or without pain. It's for every woman with a family history of breast cancer. It's for every woman whose doctor has said, "I want to check that breast again in a month." It's for every woman who wants to be more in control of her breast health, but isn't sure where to start. It's for every woman who would like to examine her breasts regularly, but doesn't know how—or who does check them faithfully, but wonders what she's feeling in there.

It's for women whose doctors are rushed and don't answer questions completely, and for women who aren't sure how to frame the questions. It's for women who are curious about *mammograms*, breast *biopsies* or *needle aspirations*. It's for women whose doctors have mentioned "fibrocystic disease" or "atypia" or "carcinoma in situ." It's for women who have undergone treatment for breast cancer and are eager to protect their remaining breast tissue. It's for women who want to keep abreast of what's happening in breast health—and who want to keep their breasts.

When there's a change in a breast, a woman has several questions: Is it cancer? Could it become cancer, or does it increase my risk of cancer? How do I get rid of the problem, or reduce the symptoms?

This book can't diagnose a specific breast problem; only a doctor can do that. But it can help answer the other questions.

A personal journey

Some women never worry about their breasts.

Growing up, they never fret about too much breast, too soon—or too little, too late. They never grow anxious about how their breasts look, or about how sexually sensitive they are. If they breastfeed their babies, they experience nary a leak nor a doubt. And they *never* agonize over a lump, a bump, a pain (or the possibility of getting them), never worry about breast cancer.

Somewhere, these women exist. I'm not one of them.

Quaking, I stood at the door to the Breast Health Center at Children's Hospital of San Francisco. My family history of breast cancer had led doctors to label me "high risk." With instructions from a pamphlet, I sometimes did breast self-examination (BSE) on my lumpy, bumpy, sometimes-painful breasts, never quite sure what I was feeling. I'd undergone a breast biopsy as a very young adult when my obstetrician discovered a lump. (No cancer, but traumatic just the same.) I had a surgeon who insisted on seeing me once a year for a breast check, but I couldn't put much trust in the rather sketchy examinations. Now I thought I felt a lump. My family doctor recommended mammograms. The film of the lumpy breast was too cloudy to show anything much; the film of the other breast showed a small cluster of *microcalcifications* (tiny calcium deposits). On the phone, my doctor simply said that this was a suspicious change and that she would send me a slip for a repeat mammogram—in four months!

As a calm, rational nurse, I realized that most breast problems are *not* cancer. *The Breast Cancer Digest* declares: "Although a variety of conditions can suggest breast cancer by producing lumps, inflammation, or nipple discharge, very few of these disorders are cancer."*

I knew that many of these symptoms come not from disease, but from normal changes in the breast; even when they do mean disease, it's usually *benign* (not cancer). Even in the case of breast cancer, the outlook is increasingly rosy. If cancer is detected early, most women survive, and they survive without the drastic surgeries of yesteryear.

So much for the rational me.

---

*National Cancer Institute, *The Breast Cancer Digest*, Second Edition, Bethesda, Maryland, 1984, p. 14.

Persuaded by the inviting newspaper advertisements, I made an appointment at the Breast Health Center. They offered a thorough breast history and examination, discussion of breast cancer risk factors, counseling on treatment for breast symptoms, and training in effective BSE. As needed, "my" nurse specialist could draw on the other specialists at the Center: a geneticist to assess individual cancer risk; a pathologist to look at breast disease, or its absence, under the microscope; a radiologist to interpret mammograms (or other tests which picture the breasts); and consulting surgeons.

I had plenty of specific questions, mostly about mammograms and microcalcifications, but I also looked forward to learning—really learning—BSE. Together, "my" nurse and I would go over every inch of breast until I gained confidence that I could identify what was normal for me.

Women are their own best lump-finders. As a nurse, I knew that about 90% of all breast lumps are found not by doctors or nurses or mammograms—but by women themselves.

The idea behind BSE is that a woman, properly trained and with the experience of regular monthly practice, will get to know her normal breasts so well that she can spot small changes; careful BSE can detect some cancers even before there's a lump to feel. Should a cancer ever develop, she will find it when it's tiny and more easily cured.

I like the viewpoint on BSE offered by Pat McCarthy, a clinical nurse specialist at the Breast Health Center: "Women come in here expecting to find disease—cancer—if they examine their breasts regularly. Our approach is different. We teach them how to *check for normal*. We want them to become familiar with their healthy, normal breasts, which will probably *always* be healthy and normal.

"Then, every month, after the slight anxiety of

checking breasts which probably haven't changed at all, women can pat themselves on the back. They know their breasts are healthy, and they can take credit for giving their breasts the very best of care. They don't have to give their breast health another thought for a month. With regular periodic checks by a health professional and routine mammograms, women can be in *control* of their breast health."

Reclaiming control

How rare that sense of control over our own breasts seems to be—and how welcome when we attain it.

We are bombarded with messages about our breasts: "Your breasts are the essence of your femininity and anything that happens to them is catastrophic." "*This* is the way your breasts should look and feel and function."

The more attention we pay to these messages, the less confidence and sense of control we have. That habit of feeling powerless and passive extends to the health care we give our breasts.

My friend Michelle, for instance, is a competent, "take charge" sort of person—except when it comes to her breasts: "The Cancer Society keeps talking about the one-in-10 women who will develop breast cancer, right? My doctor says I have fibrocystic disease, so I figure the other nine in my 'group' are the lucky ones. But what can I do about it? What will be, will be, I guess."

To look beautiful in other cultures, women have bound their feet or stretched their necks with gold bangles. In our society, *breasts* have come to symbolize what is beautiful—and feminine, soft, warm, nurturing, comforting, life-sustaining. (Some male writers portray them as engulfing and threatening as well.) Sexual partners also enjoy that soft comfort, both to look at and to feel, and they capitalize on the natural sensitivity of the breast. Our culture sees breasts as specifically sexual, a lover's province whether or not they are ever a baby's domain.

Fashion, advertising, and media industries claim breasts as their territory as well. "Feminine" and "sexy" sell products—and if there's a new twist, more products are sold. So Marilyn Monroe is glorified one moment, Twiggy the next. (When the flat-chested look is in vogue, even Venus de Milo binds her breasts and signs up for the nearest aerobics class.)

Similarly, there are fashions in breast function. One year, breastfeeding is passe; next year, every mother is breastfeeding her baby. Even the acceptable sexual responsiveness of breasts goes in cycles.

Feminist historians point to voices behind those we hear. In conservative decades, for instance, when women are "supposed" to stay home, bear children and minister to husbands, large breasts are highly valued. During periods when many women work outside the home in "masculine" jobs and when vigorous exercise is popular, smaller breasts and a more streamlined silhouette come into fashion. Author Susan Brownmiller reports that during World War I, when women wore metal corsets, the War Industries Board asked American women to give up their "armor" to release 28,000 tons of steel—enough to build and furnish two battleships.*

One recent article in a popular women's magazine listed factors influencing how a woman feels about her breasts: how well her breasts met the standards of beauty—whatever they were—while a girl was growing up; how friends and family reacted to her breasts; what lovers said about her breasts and how they treated them. They, they, they.

---

*Susan Brownmiller, *Femininity*, Linden Press/Simon & Schuster, New York, 1984, pp. 38-9.

The article did mention in passing that how a woman feels about herself (her self-image) affects how she feels about her breasts. Does she have an inner sense that she is competent, acceptable, lovable? Then she probably likes her breasts fairly well.

Pat McCarthy mentions that she's seen plenty of breasts of all varieties in her work at the Breast Health Center, and that how a woman feels about her breasts seems to have little to do with how they look. "I've seen women whose breasts didn't fit society's standards of conventional beauty—and those women thought they had the greatest breasts ever." Conversely, she's talked to women convinced their conventionally beautiful breasts were ugly.

But it's a two-way street. How a woman "sees" her breasts, her mental impression of them, is part of her body image; this, in turn, contributes to her self-image. Thus, if she doesn't believe that her breasts conform to some standard of beauty and function, her self-image suffers.

How do we reclaim our own breasts? How do we learn to establish our *own* standards of beauty and function? How do we gain (or regain) some sense of control and power over how our breasts look and feel and function—and over how healthy they are, as well?

The *first step* is to neutralize the influence of most of those breast messages.

Just who is telling us about *our* breasts—and by what right? A little anger is justified and energizing.

We broaden our perspective, distinguishing the media's spectacle of flawless, airbrushed breasts from the *real* world of real breasts. In simpler societies, where people wear few clothes, women see all kinds of breasts every day: small, massive, and in-between; pendulous, pregnant, lactating, and atrophied. Breasts receive about as much attention there as elbows do here.

(My husband, a reporter, once visited a nudist camp on assignment: "It sounded really exciting. It took about half an hour before I was taking all those uncovered breasts for granted. No more fantasy. I started wishing the women would put on sweaters.")

To help women develop a more realistic view, several breast health educators in the San Francisco Bay Area assembled a brief slide show about breasts. They wanted to demystify breasts, to show real breasts as well as "processed" ones, and to reveal the scope of breast symbolism. Various slides show photography of real breasts in women of all ages, artwork of breasts, and pictures from pornographic and popular magazines.

In a similar vein, co-authors Daphna Ayalah and Issac J. Weinstock photographed and talked to women of all ages and experiences in *Breasts: Women Speak about Their Breasts and Their Lives.** Women's groups and local breast health centers may offer other resources.

It can help to laugh at the message-givers—and at ourselves for taking them seriously. Some women authors have turned to spoof, parody, and wit to make their point: "Look, this concentration on breasts is silly. Our breasts are an important part of us, but they are not all of us. We're much more than a pair of tits!"

Step Two in reclaiming power over our breasts is not for every woman. Some women, however (especially those who are quite anxious about their breast health), find it helpful to confront mentally the *worst* possible scenario: "I could lose my breast and then die." Scary as that is, it's less terrifying when put into words than the nebulous, wordless fears that many women carry with them.

---

*Daphna Ayalah and Issac J. Weinstock, *Breasts: Women Speak about Their Breasts and Their Lives*, Summit Books, New York, 1979.

The next part of this step is imagining the *best* that can happen: "My breasts stay perfectly healthy all my life."

The final part is revising the spectrum of possibilities to reflect the presence of a consistent program of breast health care: "My breasts stay healthy, which is the most likely outcome. If I develop any problem, chances are it will be benign, because that's what most breast problems are. If by any chance I develop breast cancer, it will be found early and cured—quite possibly with a lumpectomy, which removes only a small portion of breast tissue, and radiation."

Step three: We get information. That's what this book offers, and it grew out of my own quest for accurate, up-to-date information. As we ask questions and read, we assess the qualifications of our "experts" and the validity of what they say. We need to filter everything we hear or read through the screen of our own common sense.

And our *last step* is assembling a breast care team we can trust. Since we will be checking our own breasts more often than anyone else will, we need to learn how to examine them effectively, so that we can rely on ourselves. (Some women don't feel comfortable with BSE; options for them are explored in Chapter 6.) Several organizations (the American Cancer Society, women's health or community groups, for instance) offer classes in BSE.

Finding health professionals we have confidence in is an important part of this step. We may already have a family doctor, gynecologist, internist, or surgeon who is knowledgeable and thorough in examining breasts. (Chapter 6 outlines a reasonably thorough professional breast examination.) But lack of time is the enemy, and many doctors consider a complete examination (let alone teaching) a luxury. If experienced in breast health, a nurse or nurse practitioner not only can perform a thorough examination, but may be able to spend more time teaching than the doctor can.

As we become more confident, we become more assertive, a true member of our team: "It's important to me to learn how to examine my breasts effectively. Will you teach me—or will you suggest a teacher?" "This area in this breast has changed. Would you evaluate it, please?"

For me, part of the solution was the Breast Health Center. Similar centers are springing up throughout the country, in response to women's needs and demands. Each has its own particular spirit and structure, but most combine individualized care for women with educational outreach to the community and health professionals, as well as research. (Caution: A few breast centers are strictly profit-making ventures, run by people with neither training nor credentials. As always, we need to check the qualifications and experience of those we choose as our health professionals.)

Many women come to a breast health center either on their own or after being referred by their doctor for a specific symptom (or after a cancer diagnosis when they need an expert second opinion). Anxious or panicky, they may bring a family member or friend with them, to provide moral support and to help remember information from the appointment.

Other clients do not have any specific breast complaints. Many health-conscious women see their visit as just another routine health measure—which it is.

Happily ever after?

I don't envy the women who never worry about breast cancer. A little worry is normal, reasonable, and healthy. It motivates us to find out about our breasts, protect them from potential serious problems, and learn how to deal with bothersome symptoms.

But there's worry—and then there's WORRY. That's what I was experiencing as I stood outside the door to the Breast Health Center for the first time. Did I find a "happily ever after" ending? Did I tame my anxieties, discover my problems weren't problems after all, and find freedom from breast pain?

Well, I'm "happily ever after" for *this* month. I'll think about next month when it comes.

I did learn what I should worry about, and what I could safely ignore. I learned, under the careful supervision of Cathy Coleman, "my" nurse specialist, what was normal for *my* breasts and how to examine them.

I switched surgeons until I found one who took the time to perform a reasonably thorough examination. I've been needle aspirated, biopsied, mammographed—and reassured by the results (as was Patrice by the results of her tests).

It has taken time and effort, but my doctor and I both feel that we have a fairly good idea what's going on inside those breasts. Together, we've converted nonproductive anxiety into a plan for action, harnessing that energy so that it works *for* me.

In the course of my personal journey, I've talked to breast health experts in several disciplines. From them, I've learned current information about benign breast problems, breast cancer risk factors and breast carcinoma in situ. I've discovered what mammograms and other imaging techniques can (and can't) do, and about such diagnostic techniques as needle aspirations, conventional biopsies and needle localization biopsies.

These experts have generously shared with me their access to the newest definitive research into all those breast health problems which aren't cancer. Many times, it was their own research—since these are movers and shakers in the breast health field.

It's information which needs to be passed on.

Breasts:
The Inside Story

We ask a lot of our breasts.

Month after month between puberty and menopause, the breasts must prepare for a potential pregnancy and their role of nourishing a baby. Each month, if no pregnancy occurs, the preparations are dismantled, only to begin again immediately. The breasts' only change from the cycle is pregnancy (and lactation, if the woman breastfeeds)—a variation, perhaps, but scarcely an idle interlude.

Too, in our culture we've chosen to live differently from our ancestors, and our breasts haven't had time to catch up with the changes. Human beings endure back problems because they choose to walk on two feet rather than four. Similarly, women suffer many of their breast problems as a consequence of diet, stress levels, and patterns of childbearing and breastfeeding that would astonish a cave woman.

Why learn about our breasts? If we know something about how they are constructed and how they function, we can understand better what goes wrong with them, and appreciate how much goes right. We can perform BSE more effectively if we can visualize what we're feeling. A working knowledge of breast terms also gives us a language to share with health professionals.

Physical characteristics

From the outside, the breasts of the adult female appear as a pair of mounds on the chest wall. They vary in size, shape, coloring and skin texture from woman to woman, and in the same woman at different times in her life. A network of blood vessels usually shows faintly through the skin.

In the middle of each breast is a nipple. This may protrude a little or a lot, may be on a flat plane with the breast, or may even be *inverted* (inside out)—and still be normal and functional. Nipples become stiff with cold or other stimulation, including sexual touch or a baby's suckling, because they contain spongy tissue which fills with blood and becomes taut. Even a baby's cry from the next room can trigger this stiffening, which makes it easier for a baby to find the breast and begin nursing.

Areola means "ring of color," and that's just what the pigmented area around the base of the nipple is. Nipples and areolas come in a wide range of colors, and together provide a visual bulls-eye for the hungry infant. The visible pores or tiny lumps on the areola are openings for *Montgomery's tubercles*, the sebaceous (oil) glands which lubricate nipple and areola during breastfeeding. Some women have hair around the areola, a normal variation.

What's under the skin?

The breasts include more than what fits into a bra. Breast tissue extends from the breastbone outward to the middle of the armpit, from the collarbone down to the "bra-line," and from the skin back to the pectoral (chest) muscle.

Although the breasts perch on chest muscle, they contain no muscle tissue of their own. (That's why breast "exercises" are for naught, although they may strengthen the underlying chest muscle and make the breasts appear larger.)

Each breast is divided into 15 to 20 sections, called lobes, cushioned between (and within) by fat cells which give the breast its shape and softness. The tissues which separate the sections are called *Cooper's ligaments*; they pass from the chest muscle between the lobes, and attach to the skin. These bands of strong, flexible, fibrous tissue give the breast shape and support; as they age and stretch, the breast droops.

A lacy filigree of tiny strands forms a network throughout each breast. Doctors interpreting mammograms rely on this *architecture* of fibers. They look

Drawings courtesy of The National Cancer Institute.

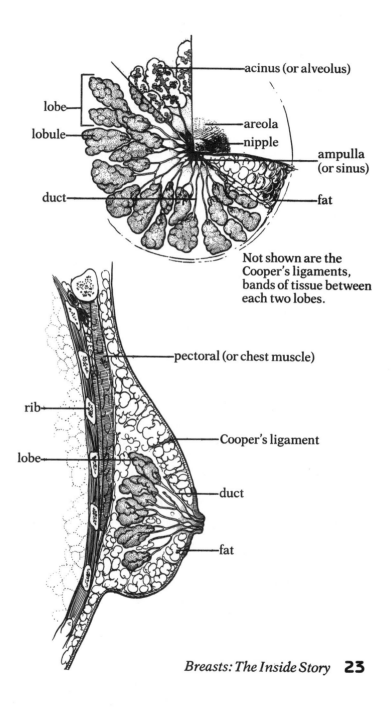

acinus (or alveolus)

lobe

lobule

areola

nipple

ampulla (or sinus)

duct

fat

Not shown are the Cooper's ligaments, bands of tissue between each two lobes.

pectoral (or chest muscle)

rib

lobe

Cooper's ligament

duct

fat

Breasts: The Inside Story **23**

for places where the network is disturbed (by a tumor, for instance), with fibers either pushed aside or unnaturally straight.

The fat cells, fibrous tissue and other parts of the breast that don't secrete or transport milk are called the stroma. The *stroma* draws wails from all the women who would prefer a little more or less breast, and can be the site of many breast problems—but rarely life-threatening ones.

The business part of the breast, the *parenchyma*, is in the lobes. Each lobe is subdivided into several *lobules*, or little lobes. Each lobule ends in several *acini* (or alveoli), tiny sacs or pockets. The minute gland cells lining each acinus are programmed by the body to extract from nearby blood vessels the ingredients they need. Like the other glands of the body, these hardworking glands recombine basic ingredients to make a particular substance; since these are mammary (or milk) glands, the substance is fluid to nourish a baby.

Providing milk

Right before and after childbirth, the gland cells follow the body's recipe for *colostrum*, a thin, yellowish fluid especially suitable for nourishing the just-born baby. After a few days, the gland cells switch to a new recipe, combining water, sugar, fat, protein, and salts in new proportions.

Once produced, the milk must travel from the gland cell to the baby. First, special cells around each acinus tighten and squeeze the fluid from the gland cells into the acinus. From each acinus, milk empties into a small *duct*. Ducts from several acini (the plural of acinus) join to form a larger channel. Milk flows through these until it reaches a reservoir, the *ampulla* or *sinus*, which ends beneath the areola. (Some people add the word *lactiferous*, or "milk-carrying"; thus ducts become lactiferous ducts, and the ampulla a lactiferous sinus.)

Milk stays dammed in the ampulla until needed. The baby's hungry cry—or the mother's imagining of a hungry cry—may signal each ampulla to "let down" or release its fluid through a pin-sized opening in the nipple. But the baby works too, both sucking milk and squeezing the ampullae (plural of ampulla) with the jaws to force out the stored milk.

The support systems

Besides the fat and fibrous tissues, which cushion and support the breast, and the gland and duct tissue which produce and transport milk, the breasts have a blood supply, lymph vessels and nodes, and sensory nerves. Blood vessels bring the breasts their basic materials for milk production, hormonal messages from the rest of the body (primarily the brain and ovaries) to perform in set ways, and the chemical energy needed for this performance.

The lymph system, the body's other circulatory system, gets rid of wastes from the breast, recycling where it can; thus, fluids and other tissues that can be reused by the body are swept into the lymph system and eventually back into the blood supply. Lymph vessels connect the two breasts and also drain each breast by way of channels through the *axilla* (armpit), along the breastbone, and up past the collarbone. Along the lymph channels are filter stations, called lymph nodes; cells that can't pass through the filters can become trapped there, most of them harmless, but an occasional one cancerous.

The nerves in the breast, concentrated in and around the nipple, provide one-way communication only. These are sensory nerves which tell the brain if they feel pressure or touch or pain. If a reply is needed, it comes in a hormonal message through the blood vessels rather than through a returning nerve. Thus, if a baby begins suckling, the breast nerves send the news to the brain, which alerts the pituitary gland in the brain, which instantly sends the hormone *prolactin* through the blood to the breast to release the milk it has stored, and to keep producing more.

The cycles

Prolactin isn't the only hormone to affect the breasts. Every month the breasts, like the uterus, gear up for a possible pregnancy. Throughout the menstrual cycle, the hormone *estrogen* flows to the breasts from the ovaries and the adrenal glands, but it reaches its peak during the middle two weeks of the cycle (counting from the first day of the menstrual period). Estrogen is the "build-up" hormone, and under its influence cells multiply and swell in preparation for possible milk production and transport. The ducts lengthen and enlarge.

When the ovary releases its ripe egg at mid-cycle, it begins releasing the hormone *progesterone* as well. This "secretory" hormone puts the prepared gland cells to work, practicing to produce milk. The blood supply increases to the breast to meet the additional needs of the working breast, and some extra fluid— basically blood minus the blood cells—seeps from the tiny blood vessels into the breast tissue. (Women may feel this as a sense of fullness, warmth, tenderness, and sometimes discomfort.)

If no pregnancy occurs, a clean-up takes place after the menstrual period. The extra fluid returns into the body's general circulation via the lymph and blood systems. The body reabsorbs unused extra cells and secretions so that the whole process can start over again. (This time of relative rest after the menstrual period—when hormonal stimulation is at its lowest— is the best time to perform BSE.)

What happens in many women over the many years of build-up/secretion/clean-up cycles is that the clean-up doesn't keep up with the build-up. The breast may receive a faulty hormonal message or may overreact to a routine message—and overprepare. Or the lymph system and other clean-up agencies may become a bit lazy on the job. Instead of being efficiently recycled, the extra fluid and secretions may gather into cysts, large or small, which persist from month to month. Only rarely do cysts become cancerous, but they do need to be evaluated (and usually drained) by a health professional.

Pregnancy and lactation

If a woman becomes pregnant, preparations for producing milk accelerate. The gland cells multiply, lobules enlarge, ducts lengthen, and blood and lymph vessels dilate. By the end of pregnancy, under the influence of estrogen, progesterone, and other hormones, the breasts have converted to a working mode, and almost all the tissue is glandular.

After pregnancy (and lactation if the woman nurses), a massive clean-up begins. The cells and structures revert to a pre-pregnant state and the lymph system scavenges the excess cells and other debris. Most of the time, this major clean-up proceeds smoothly.

Breast changes with the years

Breasts change throughout life. The rudimentary structures are present before birth, but need the starting gun of hormonal stimulation at puberty to begin growing and becoming functional.

The proportion of working or glandular tissue to the non-working stroma varies from woman to woman. But in every woman, the glandular tissue crowds out the stroma during pregnancy and lactation; fluid, rather than fat cells, gives the breast an increased size then. For a short time after pregnancy/lactation, the woman may feel that she has no breasts, as the fluid is reabsorbed and the glandular tissue recedes—until the stroma re-establishes itself.

Except during periods of pregnancy and lactation (or under the influence of certain hormone medications), the glandular tissue begins decreasing during young adulthood, slowly at first and then rapidly after menopause. Fatty tissue replaces it; in old age, the breasts are almost entirely fatty tissue.

(The dense young breast is often difficult to "image" on a mammogram; the picture appears cloudy. That's one reason why routine mammograms aren't recommended for women under 40, except for one baseline series before then. On the other hand, fatty tissue shows up clearly, which is why the films are especially useful in older women.)

Menopause, which ends the monthly hormonal rollercoaster, often spells relief from breast lumpiness and pain. Even after the ovaries have stopped functioning, however, the adrenal gland continues to supply a small amount of estrogen to regulate the fatty tissue in the older breast.

In the meantime, those lumps and bumps and sensations of fullness or discomfort are not so confusing or frightening—once we understand what's happening inside our breasts.

Lumps, Bumps, and Pains

"You have fibrocystic breast disease," declared the nurse at the University's Student Health Center as she finished examining my daughter Kathy. "Don't tell your mother about it, though. Mothers always freak out about news like that."

And for months Kathy fretted, at least a little bit, about a disease serious enough to "freak out" mothers—before she learned that she didn't have a disease at all.

What's in a name?

For years, health professionals have been labeling both lumpy breasts and lumps in breasts as "fibrocystic breast disease." It's a vague, hodgepodge term which trips nicely off the tongue, but doesn't mean much. The breast changes that doctors call fibrocystic breast disease frequently have little or nothing to do with either fibrous tissue or cysts, and often aren't disease at all. The breast is simply carrying out its normal processes, sometimes overenthusiastically.

The glandular tissue in the breast *normally* feels nodular (lumpy) during the second half of the menstrual cycle. The breast *normally* draws in extra blood and body fluid then; if there's enough to stretch the tissue and nerves, a woman may feel tenderness or pain. Some general lumpiness may remain throughout the menstrual cycle, without being abnormal, if the breasts overprepare for potential pregnancy or don't completely reabsorb the fluid afterward.

The lumpiness and/or discomfort become more pronounced in some women, perhaps because their breast tissue is more sensitive to hormonal messages, their hormonal balance is slightly out of kilter—or because their bodies are becoming older. As Pat McCarthy, clinical nurse specialist, notes, "It is common for women in their 30's to suddenly develop

Lumps, Bumps and Pains **31**

lumpy, painful breasts when their breasts had given them no problems in their 'teens and 20's."

Dr. Susan Love, Director of the Breast Clinic at the Beth Israel Hospital in Boston, estimates that half of all women have breast lumpiness that can be *palpated,* or felt with the fingers, and that even more have the microscopic changes that some doctors would diagnose as "fibrocystic disease." Why, she asks, call a common, harmless condition a disease?*

And Dr. Michael Lagios, pathologist at Children's Hospital of San Francisco, points out the crucial distinction between *detecting* breast changes and *diagnosing a disease*: "The doctor in the office can detect general lumpiness—which usually isn't a disease at all—or a specific lump. But diagnosis, finding out whether disease is present or not, takes a biopsy and a pathologist to interpret it or, in the case of a fluid-filled lump, a needle aspiration."

Fibrocystic breast disease is not only an inaccurate term, but an ambiguous one as well, because different people use it to mean different things. (This applies also to several terms used as synonyms for fibrocystic breast disease, including mammary dysplasia, fibroadenosis, chronic cystic mastitis, and mastodynia.)

Fibrocystic breast disease originally referred only to a common condition characterized by changes in the breast's fibrous tissue and the presence of fluid-filled lumps called cysts. Over the last decades, however, some doctors have broadened the term to include any benign change in the breast. Others reserve it for generalized breast lumpiness, with or without pain, without any dominant lump.

---

*Susan M. Love, Rebecca Sue Gelman, and William Silen. "Fibrocystic 'Disease' of the Breast—A nondisease," *The New England Journal of Medicine,* Vol. 307, No. 16, October 14, 1982, pp. 1010-1014.

The nomenclature wouldn't matter so much if it didn't lead to needless confusion and worry for many women. As Melanie reports: "My gynecologist felt my breasts and said, 'You have fibrocystic disease—don't worry about it.' Then my internist felt my breasts and said, 'You have fibrocystic disease and you have a higher risk of getting breast cancer.' What am I to believe?"

And the harm can be more tangible. Dr. Virginia Griswold, a radiologist, specializes in mammography and breast health. When she filled out a health form to get personal disability insurance, she sent along a copy of her health history from her own physician, including a mention of "fibrocystic breast disease." A waiver form arrived promptly from the insurance company, absolving them of financial responsibility in case of any breast disease ever.

She was astounded and furious. "I know I have no *disease* at all—but even for me, a doctor, it's an uphill road to convince the insurance company. I'm still fighting it."

Looking for answers

When a woman has a breast complaint, her first question is "Cancer?"—and her second, "Could it become cancer or does it increase my risk of cancer?" Concerned and wondering, women from all over the United States asked the American Cancer Society if they really were at increased risk for cancer with "fibrocystic breast disease." Some mentioned insurance problems. Others reported that their doctors had recommended *prophylactic*, or preventive, *mastectomies*: removing the breasts so that they wouldn't develop cancer.

ACS passed on these concerns to its National Task Force on Breast Cancer Control, which said flatly that "fibrocystic breast disease" was no longer an acceptable term, because it tarred with the same brush completely innocent normal breast processes, slight abnormalities, and a few disorders that could substantially increase a woman's risk of breast cancer. Lumping the lumps together was the real problem.

Any of the tissues or structures of the breast can react to incorrect hormonal messages or overreact to correct ones. The kind of breast change depends on what kind of tissue is involved.

Dr. Lagios, who examines biopsied breast tissue every day, compares the so-called fibrocystic breast to an overgrown garden, with all kinds of flowers and vegetables growing together. "It's true that there may be more cucumbers or roses than we'd like, but they're not causing any real problem. As a pathologist, I'm interested in only one kind of overgrowth—the radishes, for instance (in body terms, the atypical cells that can increase the risk of cancer). As long as I don't find the radishes growing wildly, I'm not concerned."

The National Task Force asked the College of American Pathologists for help in sorting out terms. In late 1985, pathologists, research scientists, and ACS representatives participated in a consensus conference entitled "Is 'Fibrocystic Disease' of the Breast Precancerous?"* (The Board of Governors of the College of American Pathologists later approved their conclusions and adopted them as policy.)

Consensus group members agreed that the term "fibrocystic disease" was inaccurate and misleading. Instead of "disease," they preferred "changes," or "condition," or "breast tissue." Better yet was "benign breast changes." These still aren't perfect,

---

*Consensus Meeting, "Is 'Fibrocystic Disease' of the Breast Precancerous," *Archives of Pathology and Labratory Medicine*, Vol. 110, March 1986, pp. 171-173.

but participants felt that creating entirely new terms at this point would only confuse matters further.

Participants also concurred that most general lumpiness doesn't need a biopsy. If a doctor calls it "fibrocystic changes," or something similar, she should clarify to the woman that this is a *normal variation* in the breast and not a disease at all. There is no increased risk of cancer.

If a biopsy is performed—for a persistent, dominant, solid lump, for certain abnormalities on a mammogram, or for any other reason—the pathologist, on finding benign changes, should define what changes. After describing the tissue, the pathologist might report, for instance, "benign breast changes: microcysts."

As Dr. Jon Ross, pathologist at Children's Hospital of San Francisco, explains: "If I report only that the tissue shows 'benign breast changes,' I'm being as precise as if I told someone to meet me 'in San Francisco.' I need to add more information, like the neighborhood and the address. Otherwise, I've just left the person dangling, without the essential facts."

The consensus group pooled their own experiences and studied all the research they could find, including the large-scale studies by William D. DuPont, Ph.D., and David L. Page, M.D., both of whom also participated in the conference. (These researchers earlier had published a landmark study reviewing over 10,000 consecutive breast biopsies by several different surgeons and pathologists at three hospitals. DuPont and Page "followed" the women for decades to see if they developed cancer after a diagnosis of benign breast disease, and drew several conclusions.*)

---

*William D. DuPont and David L. Page, "Risk Factors for Breast Cancer in Women with Proliferative Breast Disease,' *The New England Journal of Medicine*, Vol. 312, No. 3, January 17, 1985, pp. 146-151.

Participants then divided the common benign breast problems into three groups: (1) those that carry *no* increased risk for breast cancer; (2) those that increase risk *slightly*; and (3) those which increase risk *moderately*.

Breast changes with no increased risk for cancer

The consensus group found no increased risk of cancer for *non-proliferative* breast changes. Breast cells ordinarily multiply, or proliferate, to replace old cells or to prepare for pregnancy or lactation, but do so within clear limits. So when a pathologist refers to "non-proliferative" changes it means there is no cell multiplication beyond the limits of normal.

Common non-proliferative breast conditions include *fibroadenoma* (also called fibroma, adenoma, or adenofibroma, depending on the mixture of tissue in the particular lump, or tumor). This is a lump of fibrous and glandular tissue—"adeno" means gland—which is round or oval, rubbery, firm, and usually painless. It often moves freely in the breast and ordinarily occurs during the young adult years. The entire lump can be removed during a biopsy.

Breast *cysts*, whether large enough to palpate (macrocysts) or very tiny (microcysts), don't increase a woman's risk of developing breast cancer later on; in fact, some doctors believe that cysts decrease the risk of cancer. These collections of fluid or secretions can develop overnight or more slowly. They sometimes feel yielding, rather like tiny water ballons; if there's enough fluid, they can feel quite firm. Sometimes they are quite painful. Needle aspiration (see Chapter 8, p. 120) is the usual treatment for a cyst large enough to feel. The cyst collapses as the fluid is withdrawn.

Sclerosing adenosis is a common condition in which small benign solid lump(s) in the ducts of the breast are gradually replaced with cellular debris, which hardens (or scleroses). These collections of debris often calcify, which can lead to suspicious findings on a mammogram.

Other benign breast changes (see definitions in the Glossary) which don't heighten the risk of breast cancer include *apocrine metaplasia, duct ectasia,* and *mastitis* (breast inflammation). If our doctor tells us we have one of these conditions, we can relax.

Treatment? If it's a lump, it's usually removed. If it's a collection of cellular debris in the ducts—as in duct ectasia, which shows itself with a thick, sticky, grey or greenish discharge from the nipple—the involved part of the duct system can be excised (removed) by a surgeon, although often that's not necessary. Antibiotics and warm compresses cure the painful, breast infection with the kind of mastitis which not infrequently occurs in women who are breastfeeding.

Some kinds of benign breast changes which don't increase cancer risk aren't mentioned in the consensus group's list. David A. Wood, M.D., of the Cancer Research Institute of the University of California, San Francisco Medical Center (and a participant in the conference) explains that *lipoma* and *fat necrosis* are common conditions, but so obviously do not amplify cancer risk that they weren't considered by the group.

A lipoma is a clumping together of fat cells into a soft lump. Traumatic fat necrosis, generally found in older women and in women with very large breasts, usually results from an injury; sometimes it takes years after a bruise or blow for the fat in the breast to form one of these painless, firm lumps.

(Of course, some conditions are less common and haven't been studied fully. Consensus group members wanted to be *very* sure before they committed themselves to classifying a condition as one which doesn't increase the risk of breast cancer.)

The consensus group also looked at *hyperplasia*, a term which means that there are more cells than there should be, although the individual cells themselves appear to be normal. Ordinarily, the walls of the breast ducts and lobules are lined with a layer two cells deep. Participants agreed that this layer could overgrow slightly—to more than two but not more than four cells in depth—without being considered a risk factor for breast cancer.

Breast changes which increase risk slightly

If more hyperplasia develops within the lining, however, a woman's breast cancer risk rises slightly. The extra cells can be laid down either in solid layers, or in bunches that project like nipples into the ducts. This is *proliferative change without atypical cells*. This doesn't mean that the hyperplastic tissue itself is especially likely to become cancerous, but that the woman with this kind of change in her breast has a slightly greater than normal chance of developing breast cancer at some time, either in that or the other breast.

Several researchers have noted that hyperplasia often is reversible. Perhaps the breast starts responding to more appropriate hormonal messages, or the cyclic clean-up process becomes more thorough. In any case, tissue can become more or less hyperplastic, or totally normal again.

There are several varieties of *papilloma*, a benign, finger-like growth in the breast duct(s), often with a bloody or clear straw-colored nipple discharge. Only one kind—papilloma with a fibrovascular core—is clearly associated with a slight increase in risk for breast cancer; there is not yet sufficient information available about the other varieties, although they do not appear to raise the risk. The surgeon removes the involved portion of the duct system.

Breast changes which increase risk moderately

We don't exactly how and why the breast sometimes produces *atypical*, or abnormal, cells. Perhaps, if the breast is working overtime to make the extra cells of hyperplasia, the quality control slips. These atypical cells may disappear, may stay where they are without causing any trouble, or—once in a while—can lead to cancer. This *proliferative change with atypical cells* does increase a woman's risk of breast cancer moderately, whether it occurs in the ducts or the lobules.

Cells can be a little bit or a lot different from normal, just as a person can vary from the norm by being a trifle plump or 250 pounds overweight. Researchers believe that it's not only how atypical the individual cells are but also *how many* atypical cells there are that can cause problems; too many atypical cells may overwhelm body defenses that cope easily with a few such cells.

Understanding breast cancer risk

What does the American Cancer Society mean when it says, "One in 10 women will develop breast cancer"— and why does that figure seem to be increasing every few years? How much of an increase in breast cancer risk is considered "moderate"? How do factors such as family history affect breast cancer risk? Answers to questions like these fall into the bailiwick of Patricia T. Kelly, Ph.D., a medical geneticist who specializes in cancer risk analysis at Children's Hospital of San Francisco.

Lumps, Bumps and Pains **39**

Each segment of time in a woman's life carries its own small portion of risk that she will develop breast cancer. Because breast cancer is often related to body wear and tear, the risk of developing the disease increases with age: Each segment of time in a woman's life is a little riskier than the one before.

Statisticians compile *life tables* based on their current information about just how much breast cancer risk women face during each time segment throughout life (what percentage of women develop the disease during each decade of life, for instance). If the portions of risk from two or more adjoining segments of time are added together—such as risk from age 20 to 40—the result is a *cumulative risk*.

Statisticians use the life tables to predict how likely it is for a woman of a particular age to develop breast cancer during the next ten years, the next 20 years, or eventually. Eventual or *lifetime risk* is a cumulative risk figure which refers to the remainder of a female's lifetime, whether she is now a newborn infant or 90 years old.

The 10% (one-in-10) breast cancer figure cited by the American Cancer Society says that, under present conditions of risk, a white baby girl born today has a 10% chance of being diagnosed with breast cancer at some time during her life.* (The risk is slightly lower for black women.) The chances of dying of breast cancer for the same white baby girl are much lower: about 3%.

This one-in-10 breast cancer risk figure, and the rapid change from one-in-13, sound scarier than they are. What these figures reflect primarily is the rapid

---

*For 1985 ACS life table for developing breast cancer, see pp. 48-9 in Herbert Seidman, Margaret Mushinski, Steven Gelb, and Edwin Silverberg, "Probabilities of Eventually Developing or Dying of Cancer—United States, 1985," in *CA: A Cancer Journal for Clinicians*, Vol. 35, No. 1, January/February 1985, pp. 35-56.

increase in longevity for women: More women are living longer, into the decades in which breast cancer becomes more common. (Ironically, the breast cancer statistics would look much brighter if large numbers of women died young—in childbirth, for example, or of pneumonia or cervical cancer.)

The 10% breast cancer risk figure is a cumulative figure obtained by adding a woman's risk of developing breast cancer from age 20 to 30, plus that from 30 to 40, and so on. Using their life tables, statisticians have found that a woman's risk of developing breast cancer during each segment of life has remained fairly stable over the years (although some argue that it *is* becoming more common in each age group).

What has changed dramatically is how long women are living. Not long ago, 65 was considered a ripe old age; a white baby girl born today in the U.S. can expect to live into her 80's, and many much longer. (Breast cancer life tables include the years to age 110 to allow for the measurable, and increasing, group of women over 100.) This means more segments of life, each with its own portion of risk for breast cancer.

Moreover, these later decades are ones of especially high risk, simply because breast cancer becomes more common as a woman gets older. Thus, instead of a few women facing a 3% risk of developing breast cancer during a certain high-risk decade, now hundreds of thousands of women reach that decade. Those throngs of women in their 80's (at relatively high risk for breast cancer because of their age), the smaller (but growing) group in their 90's at higher risk, and the many women over 100 at highest risk all influence the statistical risk picture for the average woman. That's why the statistics have changed so quickly.

The average woman's risk of developing breast cancer from birth to age 50 is about 1.5%, notes Dr.

Kelly; from birth to age 65, the risk is about 6%, or roughly one-in-17. At no one time does the average woman face a 10% risk of developing breast cancer. She faces a small risk during each segment of time. If she does not develop breast cancer during that segment of time, that portion of risk is behind her forever. During the next segment of time, she faces another small risk.

Thinking of breast cancer risk as a series of time segments, each with its small portion of risk, becomes especially valuable when a woman has a breast problem or other factor (such as family history) which may increase her chances of developing breast cancer. Dr. Kelly stresses that, for instance, a risk factor which triples a woman's risk of developing breast cancer does not mean than she faces a 30% (3 X 10%) lifetime risk of the disease.

What *does* it mean? To calculate a woman's risk of breast cancer after a diagnosis of breast atypia at age 45, for example, Dr. Kelly would gather information about the woman and her particular atypia, and then would use analysis figures from a life table prepared by the group studying risk due to breast atypia.

Since the life table is based on the specific condition, the figures are much more precise than "moderate increase in risk." Because the risks are calculated for segments of time throughout life, the woman of 45 with atypia can find out how much risk of breast cancer a woman of her age with her particular condition faces in the immediate future, over the next several years, and over a lifetime.

For the younger years, when the average per-decade risk of developing breast cancer is very low, tripling or quintupling it still produces a relatively low—and emotionally manageable—risk. (Quintupling risk for a woman of 20 means that she has about one chance in 500 of developing breast cancer during the next decade.)

And, as Barbara says of her risk with breast atypia, "I'm not worrying much about the high risk I'll face at age 100, because I suspect that I will have dropped dead of a heart attack or something long before then. If I do make it that long, I'll have 100 years of risk behind me, anyway, so that my lifetime risk won't be much. And I wouldn't be surprised if they figure out how to prevent breast cancer by then or make a vaccine or something. I'll concern myself with now, and the next several years, but that's all."

("Slightly increased" risk was defined by the consensus conference on "fibrocystic disease" as that which raises the risk of developing breast cancer to one-and-a-half to two times the average. Conference members agreed that areas of atypia that are highly abnormal increase risk "moderately"—to about five times that of comparable women who have not undergone breast biopsy. Many clinicians would consider risk "moderately increased" when it falls between two-and-a-half and five times average risk. If they are used at all, such broad terms as "slightly" or "moderately" increased risk must be clarified for the individual woman.)

What about other factors which may increase risk of breast cancer? In evaluating family history, Dr. Kelly studies several questions: How close is the relationship? Sister, mother, aunt, or grandmother? (The relationship need not be through the mother's side to increase risk.) How old was a woman's relative when breast cancer was diagnosed? Was one breast or both affected? What type of breast cancer was it? She checks how many generations of women in the family were diagnosed with breast cancer.

After extensive data collection ("a very labor-intensive process," explains Dr. Kelly), she analyzes her information and provides a numerical risk value for the situation. In some cases, decade-by-decade risk figures are available.

A woman whose only family history of breast cancer is a mother who developed cancer in one breast at age 85, for example, may face no (or minimally) increased risk. On the other hand, a woman whose mother and sister developed breast cancer in both breasts before menopause may be at significantly increased risk for developing breast cancer also.

Some factors, such as giving birth to a first child before age 20, may decrease the risk of breast cancer. Others, such as the number of children a woman bears, don't appear to make a difference.

What about diet as an influence on breast cancer risk? Many studies point to a link between a high-fat, low-fiber diet and increased breast cancer risk; animal studies also support a connection.

Early findings (after five years) from an ongoing Harvard study of diet and breast cancer in almost 90,000 nurses initially appeared to question this link. However, the group with the *lowest* fat intake in the Harvard study consumed 32% of daily calories as fat—well below the average 42% fat intake in the U.S. diet, but still higher than fat consumption usual in countries with low breast cancer incidence. Many researchers would like to see a large-scale, long-term study of women with a fat intake of 10 to 20%. They continue to recommend major reductions of fat in the diet to reduce risk of the disease as they await further results after more years of the Harvard study.*

Many questions remain, not only about the risk of a particular element in the development of breast cancer, but also about how risks combine (atypia and a mother with bilateral breast cancer, for instance). Dr. Kelly recommends that women with specific

*Susan Rennie, "Breast Cancer Prevention: A Controversial New Diet Program," *MS.*, Vol, 15, No. 10 (April 1987), pp. 40-2, 51, 86-9. A pull-out booklet, "The Anticancer Diet Your Doctor Won't Give You," appears from pp. 43-50 of the same issue.

questions contact a cancer risk analysis program for individual assessment—and often reassurance. Medical schools or large hospitals may provide such a service, or information about locating one.

Dr. Kelly has found that many women think that their risk of breast cancer is higher than it actually is. Even when the risk is markedly increased, it's helpful for a woman to have accurate information and a perspective for that information: The unknown causes more fear than the known, she notes. With information, a woman can take appropriate steps to protect her breast health, steps such as further BSE training, more frequent checkups, prophylactic surgery and/or dietary changes.

What to do about benign breast changes

What do we do if a doctor tells us we have "fibrocystic breast disease"? We ask for clarification: "What do you mean by 'fibrocystic disease'? Do you mean the kinds of normal changes that occur in many breasts over the years?" If that's the kind of change we have, we know we don't have a health problem.

We may still have a discomfort problem (see Chapter 4). We may need additional help in learning to distinguish what's normal for our breasts during breast self-examination (see Chapter 6). However, we don't have a condition we must mention on insurance forms.

If there's a dominant lump, or other problem which requires a needle aspiration or a biopsy, we have a right to accurate, complete information about the results in terms we understand. Sometimes, a biopsy shows only mild, generalized changes without disease—tissue from normal lumpy breasts.

Pathologists say they sometimes feel pushed by surgeons, patients, or insurance companies to report breast disease even when no real disease exists.

Lumps, Bumps and Pains **45**

Surgeons believe patients will mistrust them if they've removed "normal" tissue. Some patients feel that if they have a biopsy scar, they want a disease to show for it. Insurance companies may question removal of "normal" tissue.

On the other hand, such biopsies are often necessary. Sometimes the most innocent breast changes can raise concern about cancer. The careful doctor prefers to be safe. If only breast changes that *scream* "cancer" are biopsied, many serious problems get missed until it's too late.

As health consumers, we need to understand that a breast biopsy means only that a doctor has significant questions about a breast change—questions that can be answered best by a biopsy. Of all biopsies, only a small percentage show cancer, and a few more reveal atypia. Most show normal changes or non-proliferative conditions.

Some women are reluctant to undergo biopsies because they've heard of studies showing that women who undergo biopsies for benign breast conditions have a statistically increased chance of developing breast cancer, compared to women who don't have biopsies. A closer look reveals that it isn't the fact of undergoing a biopsy that magnifies risk. Rather, it's that, out of a group of women undergoing biopsies, a few—basically those with proliferative atypias—do face more risk of breast cancer. The risk is averaged for all the women undergoing biopsies, although most of them are not at increased risk at all.

If we do have a biopsy, we need the pathologist to specify the kind of benign changes found. In cases of hyperplasia (with its slightly increased cancer risk) and atypia (with a greater increase in risk), we need to know what kind of follow-up breast health care is appropriate.

Not all doctors are up-to-date on the latest developments in breast health and disease. It takes time for new information to filter through the medical community. We, as health consumers, can help our doctors and ourselves by asking for clarification. We need to speak the same language and to understand what each other means.

What to do About Breast Pain

I used to fantasize about detachable breasts. When my breasts hurt a lot, I longed to take them off for a while. Zippers? Snaps? Velcro strips? I wasn't particular.

Once a woman is satisfied that her breast pain isn't cancer and doesn't increase her risk of cancer, she still wants to know what to do to relieve it. There's no one magic solution—but there *are* effective remedies, and virtually every woman can find one or a combination of strategies to ease discomfort. The plan involves (1) a visit to the health professional for assessment of the immediate breast problem, removal of pain-causing factors, if possible, and suggestions for treatment; (2) our own evaluation of any remaining breast pain; and (3) a trial of one or more techniques for relief of discomfort.

What the health professional can do

We visit the doctor or nurse practitioner primarily for diagnosis—to find out what a lump is or what's causing our breast pain. Happily, relief of pain can be a tag-along benefit.

Many of us equate breast pain with breast cancer, and that fear makes any pain worse. However, the fact is that pain isn't ordinarily a symptom of breast cancer. Thus, health professionals tend to be optimistic when a premenopausal woman comes in complaining of generalized breast discomfort or a painful lump, particularly when the pain and/or lump wax and wane with the menstrual cycle. Optimistic—but *not* complacent: *Any* breast complaint deserves thorough examination. Usually, after examination, the doctor or nurse can pass on reassurance, which removes the fear factor and often decreases pain.

Diagnostic procedures sometimes alleviate discomfort. A breast cyst can be quite painful. As it collapses during a needle aspiration, the pain goes.

Benign breast changes can go hand in hand with hormonal irregularities, and thus, a thorough examination for persistently painful breasts assesses the menstrual cycle and the thyroid gland for easily correctable problems.

After the examination, the health professional may be able to suggest relief measures for any residual breast discomfort.

Evaluating residual pain

If we still have breast pain, we want to know what we're dealing with in order to decide how much time and effort we're willing to devote to solving the problem. Minor problems require minor solutions; major problems call for more substantial measures.

Breast pain often disappears as mysteriously as it comes. What is agonizing in March may be gone completely in April—and ever after. Thus, if we experience occasional tenderness, or a month of bothersome discomfort once in awhile, we may decide not to treat it at all, or to use very simple remedies. On the other hand, if pain is severe, and either constant or recurring monthly, we may be willing to expend considerable energy to get rid of it.

Jotting down a few notes every day for a couple of months can be an accurate and revealing way to evaluate the problem. Our breast diary includes a brief daily note answering these questions:

What kind of pain is it? Diffuse tenderness? Dull ache? Throbbing pain? Burning sensation? Stabbing pain? Combination?

Where does it hurt? One breast or both? Localized discomfort or generalized? Does it spread beyond the breast? Near the breast surface or deep within the breast? For pain in a specific location, we can draw two circles to represent breasts, and mark the spot with an X.

When does it hurt? Does it follow a pattern, perhaps related to the menstrual cycle? (Our diary keeps track of the day of the menstrual cycle, with day one the first day of the period.) Is discomfort worse if we're feeling bored, angry, or blue? Does pain disappear some months?

How much does it hurt? How do we rate it on a scale of one to ten? Are breasts tender to touch, or painful when nothing touches them? Does discomfort wake us up, or keep us from going to sleep? Is it painful to walk or to exercise—and how painful? Do we limit our activities occasionally or regularly because of the discomfort? Does the severity change from day to day, month to month?

How and when did it begin? How long has this been going on? Did it start suddenly, with acute pain? Or did we gradually become aware that our breasts weren't as comfortable as they once were?

What accompanying symptoms are there? Swelling? Increased general lumpiness? One specific lump? Generalized bloating? Premenstrual cramping? Irritability?

The whole entry might be ten words or less, in any code or shorthand which makes sense to us, or considerably longer if we wish to make it so. What we want is a general picture of our situation. We're gathering clues, patterns, and connections which may help us and our health professionals to solve the problem. Even if no pattern reveals itself, we will be better informed participants in our own health care.

(Then again, many women discover that the

scope of their problem isn't worth the minor hassle of keeping a diary—a solution in itself.)

How we feel pain

How do we come to feel pain? Pain researchers speculate that stretching or other "injury" of nerve fibers at any site in the body releases certain chemicals. These chemicals activate a series of nerves to relay a pain message from site to spinal cord to brain. Other nerves along the spinal column may act as gates to permit or block the transmission of the pain message. Non-thinking pain perception areas in the brain receive and decode the pain message and send it on for appropriate action.

The extent of nerve fiber injury doesn't necessarily correlate with the amount of pain we feel. Plainly, what happens to the pain message *after* it leaves the injury site has much to do with our eventual perception of pain. How the gates function, and how quiet or alert the pain perception areas are, affect our feelings of pain.

We are not cookie-cutter people, each identical to the next, and each of us feels pain differently. Moreover, how we perceive pain at any time depends on the circumstances. Pain we might label excruciating at some other time may not register at all if we're sleeping, or sexually aroused, or fleeing for our lives. Other factors which affect our perception of pain include our memories of past pain, our cultural and ethnic backgrounds, and our current needs, expectations and emotions.

After the brain decodes a pain message, what kinds of appropriate action might it take? Not only can the thinking areas of the brain discover and evaluate therapies, but the non-thinking brain centers can contribute their own remedies.

Some people scoff at the idea that the brain can alleviate pain. I don't. As a nurse, I've seen many different kinds of pain, including cancer pain, relieved with a backrub, a placebo (a sugar pill or something similar), or a visit from a loved one.

We don't know yet all the factors in the brain's own pain-relieving processes. Pain researchers, however, have discovered that *endorphins* and *enkephalins* produced by the body do much the same things that morphine does—except that they do them better. They may slow or block transmission of pain messages to the brain and/or may quiet the pain perception areas in the brain. We know that sustained, brisk exercise can unleash these natural analgesics (pain-relievers); perhaps certain states of relaxation can bring a similar effect.

The discovery that the brain itself can deliver the most potent of narcotics has added a whole new dimension to the treatment of pain. It makes sense to give our brains every chance to support and bolster any pain therapy we choose.

We maximize our pain relief by expecting a treatment to work. This means keeping our minds open to reasonable therapies, using our intelligence (with a dash of skepticism) when we select a remedy, and then trusting it to be effective.

Specific remedies

To decrease breast discomfort, we must reduce the painful stimulus itself (the stretching or other irritation of nerve fibers), interfere with the transmission of the pain message from breast to brain, and/or quiet the pain perception areas in the brain. Pain relief measures include mechanical, psychological, dietary, pharmacological, and (very rarely) surgical techniques.

Mechanical measures. Many women wear a sturdy support bra, perhaps a jogging bra, 24 hours a day for relief of pain. This stabilizes and confines the breasts to reduce that stretching of nerve fibers that can trigger a pain message. Some women find it helpful to support the breasts with pillows or pads at bedtime.

On the other hand, every woman is different, and some women with breast discomfort find the touch of a support bra intolerable, so they may go braless, or wear a light bra or chemise. Some women experiment with a particular fabric against the breasts; silk, cotton, or lamb's wool may send a competing comfort message to the brain, crowding out a discomfort message at a pain gate.

A heating pad, hot water bottle, or even hands warmed in hot water and held cupping the breasts, relieve pain for some women. A hot bath or shower not only cleanses and relaxes, but can ease breast pain as well. Other women prefer cold: an ice pack or a plastic glove filled with ice, perhaps, or hands cooled in cold water and held over the breasts. Some women alternate heat and cold.

Either heat or cold can decrease swelling, each in its own way, resulting in less stretching of nerve fibers. In addition, heat and cold send their own messages to the brain, often overriding the pain message.

Massage can ease breast pain. Carolyn Gale Anderson, a certified masseuse, has worked with women and doctors to perfect techniques for easing breast pain and swelling—and she teaches women how to perform these techniques for themselves. One of her aims is to decrease swelling, and thus nerve stretching, by moving the extra tissue fluid away from the breasts along the lymph pathways.

"Women come to me with breasts that are hard and sore to touch, and with very sensitive nipples," says Ms. Anderson. "One effective technique which a woman can do at home involves soaping the breasts well in the bath or shower and then moving the fingers gently in small circles all over each breast. These circles, about the size of a coin, are like those she makes to examine her breasts.

"Then the woman can hold her hands vertically, one on each side of the breast, and press gently in and up to raise the breast. The important thing is to *move* the breasts so that the fluid doesn't just sit there.

"The relief from effective breast massage lasts about two days, and the massage can be repeated then. A woman's partner can learn these techniques too. If there's a painful cyst or hard lump, it needs to be treated by the doctor—but for generalized tenderness and lumpiness, breast massage works well."

Carolyn Anderson performs a full breast massage, including some techniques difficult for a woman to use herself, in the context of a total body massage. General massage techniques, including those as simple as rubbing our own shoulders, necks, or feet (or having someone do it for us), can send competing messages to the brain, and can quiet pain perception areas by increasing our sense of physical and psychological well-being.

Some women advocate acupressure; therapists have taught them appropriate techniques and pressure points.

Most of these mechanical therapies are free or inexpensive, readily available, and have no negative side effects. They can be very effective, without requiring major upheavals in our lives.

Psychological remedies. If the pain perception system involves the brain, so too does the pain relief process. Psychological pain relief measures include (1) those for general emotional well-being, which may actually reduce benign breast changes themselves, as well as the pain associated with them, and (2) more specific remedies for a painful episode.

Being in a relaxed state of mind—free from undue anxiety, stress, or anger—may actually decrease benign breast changes. This doesn't mean that those lumps and bumps and pains are "all in the head"; what it does mean is that our emotional state is one factor which influences our hormonal state which, in turn, affects our breasts. Many women have more general motives for improving their emotional well-being, but relief of breast problems may be a welcome bonus.

Here's where a woman's lively intelligence comes into play. Simply getting accurate information about benign breast changes should decrease breast anxiety. Counseling may be necessary for reducing other fears.

If we're alive, we have stress, and that's as it should be. Sometimes, however, we encounter more stress than we can handle comfortably, or we react to normal levels of stress in unhappy, unhealthy ways. Books, articles, classes, counseling, or discussions with health professionals can help us decrease stress, pace it better, or alter our reactions to it. Brisk physical exercise, relaxation training, with an emphasis on breathing patterns and alternate tensing and relaxation of muscle groups, and meditation are techniques for managing stress. Sometimes, a job or relationship change may be indicated.

Sometimes, we unconsciously cling to pain because it seems better than the alternative or it brings us some benefits. It may make others sympathetic, for instance, or save us from shouldering some responsibility we'd rather avoid.

Along with tossing out our negative emotional baggage, we want to bring aboard all the positives we can find: laughter, involvement, relaxation, commitment. Finding something really fascinating to do is a marvelous cure for all sorts of ills. That something fascinating can be a relationship, a job, a hobby, or something entirely different. One woman may find it in prayer, another in gardening, raising a child, writing a journal, or carrying out a research project.

As a nurse, I constantly use specific psychological pain relief measures—especially distraction, relaxation techniques, and visualization—for patients, including myself, experiencing any kind of pain. Distraction simply means taking one's mind off pain by focusing on something else, preferably something absorbing. This quiets the pain perception center so that it's less ready to accept pain messages. (Some women do the opposite, focusing closely on the discomfort, until they "work through it" and it doesn't bother them any more.)

The body stops perceiving many pain messages when it's asleep, in a state of profound relaxation. The closer we get to that degree of relaxation, the less pain we experience. Thus relaxation techniques, helpful in managing general stress, can be called into play also during specific episodes of pain.

Some women become adept at a variety of visualization techniques—from "seeing" themselves in some very inviting setting (on a beach, perhaps, with sand warming and cradling their breasts), to visualizing the swelling or lumpiness leaving their breasts as fluid is reabsorbed. Classes and books can help perfect visualization techniques.

Overall, psychological therapies aren't as simple as an ice pack or a support bra. On the other hand, for many women they can deliver impressive dividends in general well-being, as well as long-term improvement in breast health.

Dietary therapies. For a seriously overweight woman, losing weight makes sense for general health; it may also relieve breast pain and lumpiness.

Reducing salt in the diet, especially during the second half of the menstrual cycle, may decrease the breasts' tendency to retain fluid and swell. Many women find this a relatively simple and effective measure.

In the late 1970's, health professionals interviewing women reported that a significantly high percentage of those with benign breast lumpiness and pain were heavy consumers of coffee, tea, chocolate, and/or cola beverages. Researchers made a scientific guess that *methylxanthines*, chemical substances found in all these products, might be a culprit in benign breast problems; caffeine is the most common methylxanthine.

The physiologic reasoning went like this: Researchers found increased levels of specific chemicals (collectively called cyclic AMP) in women with "fibrocystic" changes, but not in women without such changes. Methylxanthines tend to slow or block the action of these chemicals in the body. Thus, instead of being used up quickly, the chemicals linger in the body and may build up in the breasts, possibly leading to lumpiness and pain.

Several research projects have attempted to prove or disprove this scientific guess. The simplest studies simply asked women with breast lumpiness and pain to avoid methylxanthines for several months and report the results. Both patients and researchers expected the treatment to work—and it did.

Later studies added a *control group*, a group which would maintain its regular diet, to compare with the *treatment group*. Results were much less clear, since members of both groups improved. Researchers ascribed this finding to the unpredictable course of benign breast disease, which often comes and goes without apparent rhyme or reason.

A study of about 3400 women failed to show a link between methylxanthine comsumption and any kind of benign breast change or tenderness.* Researchers for the study also reported the findings of other investigators that cells treated with caffeine *don't* accumulate cyclic AMP, and that levels of methylxanthines normally consumed by humans are much too small to influence cyclic AMP levels.

However, many women claim they have decreased pain and lumpiness when they restrict methylxanthines in their diet. Some women may have increased sensitivity to methylxanthines—or there may be some connection we haven't discovered yet.

Reducing or eliminating methylxanthines (caffeine, theophylline, and theobromin) may be worth a serious try for the woman whose diet is high in these substances. Incidentally, caffeine appears even in many decaffeinated products, though in lesser amounts, and is a common component of pain medications which combine two or more ingredients. (Ingredient lists can be checked for the presence of caffeine.)

Both the nutritionists and the pharmacologists lay claim to the vitamins, minerals, trace elements and fatty acids that figure in several remedies for breast complaints.

The rationale behind many vitamin therapies has to do with the effect of the individual vitamin's influence on the comings and goings of estrogen in the body. Vitamin A, for instance, can inhibit the production of estrogen, and some researchers report decrease of pain and lumpiness when women increase their consumption of Vitamin A.

Vitamin B1 helps the liver metabolize estrogens, and a deficiency increases sensitivity to pain. All the B vitamins have sometimes been grouped as "stress

---

*Catherine Schairer, Louise A. Brinton, and Robert N. Hoover, "Methylxanthines and Benign Breast Disease," *American Journal of Epidemiology*, Vol. 124, No. 4, October 1986, pp. 603-11.

vitamins," and several thoughtful health professionals believe that we need more of them than our daily diet ordinarily provides, to counteract some of the negative effects of unremitting tension on the body. They reason that life styles have changed faster than the body's mechanisms for using nutrients, with the result that our diets lag in meeting our requirements.

Vitamin E affects the interplay of the reproductive hormones. As with the methylxanthine studies, results of research have been conflicting.

Very high doses of vitamins can produce negative side effects. When the vitamin is a fat-soluble one (like vitamins A, D, and E), too much can be poisonous, since the body doesn't get rid of excessive doses easily. For benign breast changes, common suggested daily doses are 5000 I.U. Vitamin A, 100 mg Vitamin B1, and 200-800 I.U. Vitamin E. Since large amounts of Vitamin E can raise blood cholesterol levels, medical monitoring is advisable.

Studies in both animals and women suggest that breast lumpiness and pain may be linked to a deficiency of iodine in the diet—and can be treated successfully by adding iodine, especially in its elemental form. Canadian and U.S. researchers, working together, report that cysts, areas of fibrosis, and breast pain have disappeared in about three fourths of women treated with 3-6 mg of elemental iodine daily, and have improved markedly in most of the other women. Several women in the study of over 300 women had an increase of pain for one to three weeks shortly after treatment started, but no pain thereafter. Tests of treatment with other forms of iodine began in 1982, with elemental iodine more recently.*

---

*Research by William R. Ghent, and B. A. Eskin, reported by Ellen Russ, "Iodine Replacement Effective in Treating Fibrocystic Disease," *Oncology Times*, January 1, 1987.

Studies in Britain recommend dietary supplementation with essential fatty acids to treat benign breast changes. Oil of the evening primrose (along with Vitamin C) provided the essential fatty acids in the clinical trials.

Researchers throughout the world are testing various vitamins, minerals, herbal remedies, and dietary manipulations for their effects on benign breast lumpiness and pain. Their medical and nutritional detective work may well bring us the relief we seek.

Pharmacological remedies. Medications used for relief of benign breast discomfort include pain-relievers, diuretics, hormones, and anti-hormones. For occasional mild-to-moderate pain, many women take aspirin or non-aspirin analgesics. (If they're restricting methylxanthines in the diet, they should avoid pain-relievers with caffeine listed among the ingredients.)

Some women ease breast pain by using *diuretics* ("water pills") and restricting salt to reduce breast swelling. Many diuretics also deplete the body's store of potassium; extra orange juice or a banana in the diet are easy ways to replace the potassium.

Women with breast problems related to *hypothyroidism* (under-active thyroid gland) often find dramatic relief from their breast troubles when they start taking thyroid hormone. Some researchers have reported decreased breast lumpiness and pain when they tried doses of thyroid hormone on women with low-normal levels of thyroid function. Since the thyroid gland uses iodine for its work, the research studies on supplemental thyroid hormone and elemental iodine—each used to decrease breast swelling, lumpiness and pain—may intersect eventually.

Oral contraceptives (birth control pills) decrease lumpiness and/or pain for many women, often after an initial period of increased tenderness. By stopping ovulation, these provide the breasts with a change comparable to the one they get during pregnancy. Thus, if a woman and her doctor agree that birth control pills are the best method of contraception for her, she may enjoy freedom from breast pain as a welcome side benefit.

Unfortunately, benign breast problems often begin when a woman is in her 30's or 40's when the health risks of taking "The Pill" multiply, especially for women who smoke. In fact, some manufacturers recommend that estrogen/progesterone pills be taken with caution by women with benign breast changes.

Sometimes estrogen-only pills bring improvement, and sometimes they make the problem worse, while bringing their own risks and side effects. So too for progesterone pills.

For very severe cases of benign breast problems, some doctors prescribe *danazol* (brand names include Danocrine and Cyclomen), a synthetic male sex hormone. Usually given for two to six months without interruption, danazol appears to be quite effective, and is especially useful in decreasing some of the benign lumps that lead to repeated biopsies. Unfortunately, danazol commonly is linked to such side effects as growth of facial hair, thickening of body hair, weight gain, decrease in breast size, acne, and oiliness of skin and hair. (Some women don't suffer any of these side effects, and some others experience them very mildly.) Danazol is also expensive. It is an option for the woman with severe breast symptoms.

Some researchers have tried *tamoxifen citrate* (Nolvadex), which interrupts estrogen's function in the body, for severe breast pain and/or lumpiness. Another prescription compound, *bromocryptine* (Parlodel), inhibits the secretion of the hormone prolactin and often improves benign symptoms. However, neither tamoxifen nor bromocryptine has been officially approved yet for use in treating benign breast changes. These potent drugs haven't been studied long enough to demonstrate the long-term effects. Most researchers agree that they should be reserved for unusually severe and persistent pain and should be given for the shortest possible periods.

Surgical treatment. If a woman continues to have severe breast pain, some doctors recommend removing the breast tissue under the skin and replacing it with sacs of silicone gel. In the case of a woman with extreme pain *and* repeated biopsies showing atypical cells *and* a strong family history of breast cancer, this is a reasonable choice. For pain alone, it's usually an excessive treatment.

For a woman contemplating this kind of surgical treatment, two or more outside opinions from doctors who would not be involved in the surgical procedure should be mandatory (including one from a specialized Breast Clinic, if possible). This is not something to undergo lightly.

Breast pain is no joke. It can be an occasional nuisance—or a continuing misery.

But there's good news about breast pain, as well: (1) It usually does not mean breast cancer; (2) most discomfort can be vanquished with careful use of appropriate remedies; and (3) even the most recalcitrant pain will disappear eventually, with pregnancy, lactation, or menopause—or simply because this is *this* month, and not last month.

When the Diagnosis is Breast Carcinoma In Situ

The way Elizabeth tells it, she didn't know there was such a thing as breast carcinoma in situ—until her doctor told her she had it.

"I had never had the slightest bit of trouble with my breasts," she recalls. "No lumps. No pains. My friends were always complaining about their breasts, but I never had any problems."

When she was 42, Elizabeth had a routine mammogram. It was normal except for a cluster of white specks of calcium salts—microscopic *calcifications* (also called *microcalcifications*)—in an area of one breast.

In many cases, a radiologist can be reasonably certain that the microcalcifications are innocent ones, associated with benign breast changes. In Elizabeth's case, however, the radiologist was more concerned. Because of the appearance of the individual specks and their clustering, there was a strong possibility that these microcalcifications could be a sign (in this case, the only sign) of more serious trouble. Like a breast lump, the microcalcifications could signal any one of many things, from the most benign of breast changes to *invasive* ductal breast cancer (in which cancer cells have broken through the walls of the breast ducts to penetrate or "invade" surrounding tissues).

The radiologist recommended that Elizabeth have a biopsy and Elizabeth's physician sent her to a surgeon. Because the abnormality was a mammogram finding rather than something that could be felt with the fingers, the surgeon collaborated with the radiologist to perform a needle localization biopsy (see Chapter 8, p. 126). On microscopic examination, the pathologist found a small area of highly atypical cells in an abnormal arrangement, confined to a duct of the breast: *duct* (or ductal) *carcinoma in situ* (DCIS, also called noninvasive or noninfiltrating ductal carcinoma).

Duct carcinoma in situ

"When my surgeon told me I had duct carcinoma in situ—whatever that meant—I just went numb," Elizabeth remembers. "I knew that carcinoma was another name for cancer, and that's all I heard, that and 'mastectomy.' I didn't faint or anything, but nothing much registered."

Until recently, surgeons routinely recommended a total mastectomy for patients with duct carcinoma in situ. Aware that new studies on DCIS were beginning to emerge, however, Elizabeth's surgeon suggested that she seek a second opinion at the nearby Breast Health Center at Children's Hospital of San Francisco.

"I called the Breast Health Center the next day," says Elizabeth. "I hadn't slept much. I was still in a fog, except for an occasional lightning attack of panic. My husband, Mike, wasn't in much better shape. He had only my disjointed report to go by since he hadn't been able to talk to the surgeon yet."

By phone, the nurse specialist at the Breast Health Center assured Elizabeth that her confused blur of feelings was absolutely normal and offered her a little more information (although Elizabeth still couldn't assimilate much). Then the nurse began the process of obtaining Elizabeth's pathology report, biopsy slides and mammograms, and of setting up consultations with the breast care team members. She urged Elizabeth to bring her husband or a friend with her, if possible, to act as a support person to listen, write down notes and questions, and just *be there*. (If no family member or friend had been available to accompany Elizabeth, the nurse would have acted as the support person.)

At Children's Hospital, the radiologist re-examined Elizabeth's mammograms, the pathologist reviewed the slides from the biopsy, the geneticist meticulously reviewed her family history and breast cancer risk factors, and a surgeon palpated her breasts to find out how easy they were to examine. Meanwhile, Elizabeth and Mike learned more about DCIS.

"The first thing we learned," recollects Mike, "was that the 'in situ' part of Elizabeth's diagnosis was very significant. It meant that the abnormal cells were confined to their original site in the duct of the breast, that they hadn't broken through the duct walls. Doctors used to consider carcinoma in situ as just an early cancer, something that would inevitably spread if you gave it enough time. But now the thinking about it is beginning to change—although the name hasn't changed yet."

Doctors know that atypical cells in the breast increase the risk of developing cancer, and that the more atypical the individual cells are and the more of them there are, the higher the risk becomes. That doesn't mean that every atypical cell—a cell that is irregular in shape, different in internal organization, or strange in behavior—will become cancer if left long enough. (In fact, the body probably disposes of some atypical cells, including cancer cells, all the time, through its defense systems or during the normal turnover of cells.)

But atypical cells are more likely than normal cells to pass on their strangeness as they divide, so that succeeding daughter cells are similarly, or even more atypical. Thus, breasts which tend to form large numbers of atypical cells are more likely to form threatening numbers of the most atypical cells: cancer cells.

Pathologists grade atypical cells by how unusual they are. Grade 1 on the continuum refers to cells which look only a little bit different from normal cells; grades 6 and above mean cells so bizarre in appearance and arrangement that they must be considered cancerous. These grades are not neat pigeonholes, however, and pathologists sometimes disagree about how a particular biopsy specimen should be classified.

Grade 5 cells are carcinoma in situ. By definition, "in situ" means that while the problem cells may push neighboring breast tissue out of the way, they have neither penetrated adjacent breast structures (as in invasive cancer) nor spread beyond the breast (as in metastatic cancer).

There is usually no lump or anything else to palpate with DCIS, but it often leaves telltale "fingerprints"—microcalcifications on mammograms—to show its presence. Until mammography came of age, DCIS was ordinarily discovered only by accident, when the highly atypical cells were found in tissue that had been biopsied for some other reason. Prodded by mammographers, however, surgeons began to hunt for DCIS, performing breast biopsies when the sole abnormality found before the tissue sampling was a cluster of microcalcifications on the mammogram.

By the early 1970's, surgeons and pathologists were seeing large numbers of women with DCIS. Doctors acknowledged that the in situ cells did not act like the rampaging cells of invasive cancer—yet—but their only question was "how soon will they invade or metastasize?" Total mastectomy was the treatment.

For Dr. Philip Westdahl, surgeon at Children's Hospital of San Francisco, a mastectomy he performed for DCIS in July of 1972 marked a turning point in his thinking. "I felt that the biopsy had removed the DCIS, an area no more than a few millimeters in diameter with a clear margin of normal breast tisssue around it—and, from all the evidence, the DCIS was gone. These cells didn't penetrate into the adjacent breast tissue. Why should I have to remove the entire breast? It seemed to me that mastectomy in such cases went way overboard."

He shared his concern with Dr. Michael Lagios, a pathologist at Children's Hospital. Intrigued, Dr. Lagios began to re-examine in painstaking detail all the cases he could find where a breast had been removed for a diagnosis of DCIS. As he expected, he found that microscope slides from the breasts sometimes contained evidence of invasive cancer. However, he couldn't discover any traces of invasive cancer in breasts in which the area of DCIS was less than 25 millimeters (about one inch) in its largest diameter. In breasts with areas of DCIS larger that 25 millimeters, Dr. Lagios found that the larger the area, the greater the chance of invasive breast cancer. DCIS was occasionally *multicentric*, with clusters of cells elsewhere in the same breast, but if one area of DCIS revealed itself with microcalcifications on a mammogram, so did the other areas.

Drs. Lagios and Westdahl began to view DCIS as the last stage of benign breast changes—a very abnormal benign atypia—rather than as the first stage of breast cancer. As such, it is not "biologically committed"; that is, several different outcomes are still possible. Like the other benign atypias, it may be reversible, regressing with the normal turnover of cells in the body, or it may stay unchanged. In some cases, it may change into an invasive cancer.

Drs. Westdahl and Lagios did not doubt that areas of DCIS should be taken out of the breast along with an adequate margin (border) of normal breast tissue—but did the entire breast have to be removed too? By 1974, they felt ready to recommend another option to a carefully selected group of highly motivated women with DCIS.

The area of DCIS itself, along with a margin of normal breast tissue around it, would be removed, and the specimen subjected to careful examination by both radiologist and pathologist to be sure that all the microcalcifications and DCIS were included in the specimen; if microcalcifications or DCIS cells were found at or near the edges of the specimen, more tissue was removed from the breast until the margin contained only normal breast tissue. (There was no reason to sample tissue from the lymph nodes, since DCIS, by definition, had not metastasized.) Then the woman would have follow-up examinations every three months by the surgeon, and a yearly mammogram to check for any new cluster of suspicious calcifications or a lump too small to palpate.

It made sense, but it marked a departure from the standard treatment for DCIS. The doctors realized that accepting this treatment option would require understanding and faith on the part of both patient and doctor.

They set up a protocol with stringent criteria (which they still follow):* The area of DCIS must be less than 25 millimeters in its largest diameter, preferably smaller. It has to show itself by microcalcifications on a mammogram. It cannot contain any trace of invasive cancer on microscopic interpretation by the pathologist.

The woman's breasts must be easy to examine, so that any new DCIS or invasive cancer can be detected promptly. Thus, they can't have cysts or major background lumpiness that could conceal a small cancerous lump from the examining hands of the surgeon. Also, the breast tissue must image clearly on a mammogram, to catch early any new microcalcifications or a tiny lump. (This excludes women with very dense breasts which are difficult to mammograph accurately.)

---

*Michael D. Lagios, "Human Breast Precancer: Current Status," *Cancer Surveys*, Vol. 2, No. 3, 1983, pp. 384-401.

The woman cannot have other major risk factors for breast cancer. Usually this means a family history of a close relative with premenopausal and/or bilateral breast cancer. (Now all patients considering this treatment option are evaluated by Dr. Patricia T. Kelly, the medical geneticist at Children's Hospital who specializes in cancer risk analysis.)

In addition, the woman must be fully informed of the risks involved, must understand them, and must accept them.

What are the risks? Total mastectomy offers a 100% cure rate, at the cost of a breast. (There is no guarantee against breast cancer in the other breast, however.)

The minimal treatment option—removal of the area and meticulous follow-up care—leaves the woman at some risk for developing new areas of DCIS or invasive breast cancer. The woman with any atypia faces a significant risk of subsequent breast cancer (see Chapter 3, "Understanding breast cancer risk," pp. 39-45); the more abnormal the atypia, the higher the risk. The average risk of getting invasive breast cancer for a woman with DCIS is about *1% each year*.

Elizabeth continues: "What the doctors stressed was that I had to feel comfortable with my decision. If I couldn't sleep nights worrying about the possibility of cancer, mastectomy would be a wiser choice. However, if I really wanted to keep my breast, and was willing to go through all those exams to do it, this was a reasonable option with an acceptable risk.

"If they should find another tiny area of microcalcifications and it's DCIS, they can do the same procedure again. If they ever find an area of invasive cancer, it will be small and I would still have the options of mastectomy or possible lumpectomy with radiation. Or if I change my mind for *any* reason, I could still have a mastectomy.

"I've been in the protocol some time now. I feel very lucky that I had this choice."

Not all physicians agree that this minimal treatment option is adequate for DCIS. "Initially, one surgeon called us dangerous," Dr. Westdahl admits. "All I can say is that in this carefully selected group, followed with a stringent protocol, the results over the 12 years of the study have been very encouraging. We feel they justify continuation of our method of treatment."

Some doctors prescribe radiation to the breast after a biopsy for DCIS because of the possiblity that other areas might contain invasive cells. Drs. Westdahl and Lagios and their team don't, because they believe it's unnecessary for the small areas of DCIS they are treating. In addition, they want to keep radiation as an ace in the hole in case it's needed for a subsequent invasive cancer of any type in either breast; the amount of radiation a woman can receive safely is limited.

Lobular carcinoma in situ

DCIS isn't the only form of breast carcinoma in situ. The other types are *lobular carcinoma in situ* (LCIS or lobular neoplasia) and Paget's disease of the nipple.

If DCIS is the radiologist's disease, lobular carcinoma in situ is the pathologist's. LCIS doesn't usually reveal itself with either a lump or microcalcifications; instead, it's discovered by the pathologist incidental to a breast biopsy for some other problem.

Like DCIS, lobular carcinoma in situ tends to show up in premenopausal women. Despite its name, LCIS is found, like DCIS, in the terminal ducts of the breast lobules. Also like DCIS, lobular carcinoma in situ puts women at increased risk of developing invasive breast cancer later, though it does not itself penetrate neighboring tissues or spread beyond the breast.

Unlike DCIS, however, which typically is confined to one breast, lobular neoplasia is usually found in both breasts; even if it's not in both breasts yet, both breasts are at equal risk for developing new areas of lobular neoplasia. Also unlike DCIS, the size and numbers of areas of lobular neoplasia don't appear to affect the prognosis: Widespread LCIS is no more likely than a tiny area to be associated with invasive breast cancer.

The traditional treatment for lobular neoplasia has been removal of the breast in which it was found, along with a biopsy of the opposite breast. That didn't make sense to many doctors. With no lump or micro-calcifications as a guide for selecting the tissue to biopsy from the second breast, finding lobular neoplasia would be a matter of blind luck. Both breasts should be removed—or neither breast.

A team of doctors at the Laboratory of Surgical Pathology at Columbia University in New York noticed that of those women who did not have any treatment beyond the original biopsy, few developed invasive breast cancer. (These were cases in which the pathologist missed seeing the neoplasia or the women refused mastectomy for some reason.)

The alternative offered by doctors at Columbia and at Children's Hospital of San Francisco is similar to that for DCIS: If lobular neoplasia without any invasive cancer is found during examination of breast tissue after a biopsy, no additional surgery is per-formed; there are follow-up examinations every three to four months, with less emphasis on mammography than during follow-up for DCIS. The goal is to find any invasive cancer, as evidenced by a tiny lump, at the earliest possible moment.

The invasive cancers associated with lobular neo-plasia tend to be "lazier" forms of the disease—rela-tively slow-growing, slow-spreading tumors. According to Dr. Kelly, the actual risk of developing invasive breast cancer after a diagnosis of LCIS (based on a study of over 250 women) is 16% during the first 20 years, or a little less than 1% each year.

Dr. C. D. Haagensen of Columbia Medical Center has been offering this option to women with lobular neoplasia for over 30 years. He states, in his *Diseases of the Breast*, that "no patient of mine with lobular neoplasia who has returned regularly every four months for examination has lost her life."*

Paget's disease of the nipple

Very few women develop *Paget's disease of the nipple*. When it does occur, it shows itself first as an eczema-like rash on and around the nipple.

Doctors long considered Paget's disease of the nipple a "beachhead" established by an underlying breast cancer. Dr. Lagios, however, noted that breasts removed for Paget's disease of the nipple often contained *no* evidence of invasive breast cancer. He looked, too, at breasts in which the disease had been misdiagnosed for years as eczema, but had not progressed.

He concluded that Paget's disease of the nipple, like Paget's disease elswhere in the body, is an "in situ" change, which isn't cancerous in itself, but does significantly increase a woman's risk of invasive breast cancer later.

Since the lesion is rare, research studies have involved only a few women. For several years, Dr. Lagios has followed five women who had only the nipple and the area under it removed for Paget's disease of the nipple, and where there was no evidence at surgery of invasion of deeper breast tissue. To date, none

---

*C. D. Haagensen, *Diseases of the Breast*, Third edition, W. B. Saunders company, Philadelphia, 1986, p. 240.

of the women has shown any signs of developing invasive breast cancer.

What does it mean for us?

Throughout the field of breast health care, there's a move toward less drastic treatment. With in situ breast changes, as with tiny invasive cancers, the trend is toward preserving the breast—when it can be done with "reasonable" safety. But there's plenty we don't know yet, and what seems reasonable safety to one woman may seem intolerable risk to another.

In any case, if a woman has an in situ breast problem diagnosed, it makes sense for her to get all the information she can before she and her doctors *together* make a decision about treatment. Doctors contribute their own expertise and their reading of current medical literature. The hospital or community may provide a breast consultative service, or a "tumor board" where doctors can discuss treatment options. In addition, doctors can obtain new research findings through computerized information systems like PDQ (from the National Cancer Institute), with access terminals in many hospitals, medical libraries, and cancer centers.

What's the woman's role in this process? If there appear to be choices in treatment, a second opinion is advisable. A hospital-based breast health center is an obvious resource, for information and for referrals to physicians. Besides getting information, however, the woman must consult her own feelings, her own past ways of dealing with life, and her own priorities.

Some women are worriers; some aren't. Some women are comfortable with risk-taking; some aren't. Some women place a very high value on how their breasts look; others don't care so much. *Many* women are more resilient than they think they are, and will respond well emotionally whatever the choice.

The idea is to find a treatment plan that a woman and her doctors can accept. For a woman with DCIS, a family history of breast cancer, and breasts difficult to examine, this may mean removing the breast tissue and replacing it with a sac of silicone gel.

Or one of the minimal treatment options may be appropriate for both the physical condition and a woman's emotional makeup. Whatever she and her doctors choose, they want something they can live with happily—for many decades to come.

Examining
the Breasts

When it comes to detecting breast problems early, I want *experts:*

1. A skilled mammography team—radiologist and technician—with a method that can detect some breast changes before they can be felt;
2. A careful doctor or nurse to perform regular professional breast examinations based on experience with many different breasts;
3. Myself—the expert on my breasts, with fingers, eyes, and brain trained through many breast self-examinations.

No *one* method of detection is perfect, but mammography, professional breast examination, and BSE work *together* as a near-perfect team. Each method finds certain breast changes that the others can miss; each has particular advantages and weaknesses. The woman who uses all three methods gives herself the best obtainable breast health care.

Breast self-examination

What particular advantages does BSE offer? BSE involves the person most concerned with her own breasts and potentially most familiar with them. It provides the most constant surveillance of the breasts, since health professionals and mammograms rarely check breasts every month. BSE is free, and a woman doesn't have to leave home for it. In addition, it's available to the woman who's too young for routine mammograms.

So why don't more women use it? They offer plenty of reasons:

1. "I don't think it really makes any difference." "If there's any problem, my doctor will find it," says

Beth. "Plus I get mammograms every few years. That should be enough."

More than 90% of all breast lumps are first discovered by the woman herself, rather than by a doctor or a mammogram. However, too many of these are discovered by chance, when they are relatively large; in contrast, a lump detected through conscientious monthly BSE is ordinarily very tiny. The difference between living and dying after a diagnosis of breast cancer is usually how early the disease is detected, diagnosed, and treated. In addition, the "minimal treatment options" which preserve the breast (like lumpectomy with radiation) are available only to those with small tumors.

If a woman has a professional breast examination every March, for instance, and a cancerous tumor becomes large enough to be felt in April, she has lost 11 crucial months before the change is detected by her doctor the following March—unless she performs regular BSE. Mammography finds *many* early changes in *many* women, but misses some cancers completely.

Numerous studies show that women find any breast cancer earlier if they perform BSE regularly, and that they live longer and may save their breasts as well as a result. Until medical science learns how to prevent breast cancer, the best strategy is finding it early if it should occur. That means BSE.

2. "I don't feel competent to perform BSE. Everything feels lumpy to me."

"I'd be willing to examine my breasts regularly if I had some idea of what I was supposed to be feeling for," claims Veronica. "I tried it once and just fumbled around. It's a waste of time for me."

Women lack confidence because they haven't been trained in BSE, haven't done it long enough to develop confidence, and/or expect too much of themselves. Women need instruction, and preferably guided practice to learn the skill of effective BSE.

Finding what to look for during visual inspection of the breasts, and what parts of the fingers to use in what patterns, can come from a book or pamphlet. It's more difficult for a woman to learn what's normal for *her* breasts from a pamphlet. Guidance from a doctor or nurse has saved many a woman from panicking when she discovers a large, hard lump—which happens to be the tip of a rib.

No woman is competent at first. It takes time to "learn" the breasts. For the first few months, especially with the lumpy breasts that most young women have, everyone wonders if this particular finding is really new this month, or just escaped notice last month. That's the natural process of learning. Each month brings increasing proficiency and confidence, *if* women don't get discouraged and give up too soon.

The *only* conclusion a woman needs to draw after a self-exam is whether her breasts have changed or not since the last exam. No woman has to interpret or diagnose what any change means; that's the doctor's job. Nor does she have to be 100% sure that this *is* a change. If she *thinks* she sees or feels something different from last month, it's time to check with her health professional.

3. "I don't have time for BSE." BSE takes only 15-20 minutes of unhurried time each month. Some of the examination can be done during a bath or shower, or while drying afterwards. It's a minor time investment for a major breast health dividend.

4. "I'm scared of what I'll find." Every woman is scared that she'll find something; it's a natural fear. However, even should a woman discover a breast lump at some time, chances are that it will be benign.

With the stakes as high as they are—lives and

breasts—it's worth disregarding the fear and performing BSE anyway. And, indeed, the emphasis of BSE should be on *checking for normal*, as women assure themselves that their breasts, once again, have not changed since last month.

5. "I feel uncomfortable touching my breasts and looking carefully at them." If a woman doesn't like the way her breasts look, it *is* hard to examine them carefully. Some of the techniques for reclaiming control over the breasts (Chapter 1, pp. 13) can be helpful.

Many women grew up believing that touching or looking carefully at their bodies was wrong, and it is difficult to overcome these feelings. Slow desensitization may work: touching the breasts lightly at first, or through material, for instance, with further steps later. (For the woman who remains uncomfortable touching her breasts, "Who should perform BSE," below, can be useful.)

There are plenty of reasons for not doing BSE. For years, I had a mental quiverful of them as I bumbled through occasional, half-hearted self-examinations. Once I learned how to perform *effective* BSE, however, and gradually gained confidence that my fingers and eyes and brain could make a significant difference in my breast health, the reasons *for* performing BSE crowded out the others.

I like the peace of mind that regular BSE brings.

Who should perform BSE? Some doctors believe girls should start practicing BSE as soon as there's breast tissue to feel, at the time of the first menstrual cycle, as part of the experience of becoming a woman. The American Cancer Society recommends age 20. Other health professionals argue that, since breast cancer is so rare in women under 25, BSE is a waste of time before that.

Many women didn't hear about BSE when they started menstruating, and maybe not at age 25 either. In that case, *now* is a good time to start. (However, some women may want their adolescent daughters to become aware of BSE—and comfortable with it—as a strategy for keeping themselves healthy.)

While BSE technically means that a woman examines herself, there are alternatives. What is important is that the breasts are examined regularly and often by someone who is familiar with them. For the woman who has difficulty examining herself, for any reason, her spouse or partner can perform the exam. A health professional can examine the breasts often, although that entails the woman's traveling to the health facility and paying fees. (Some facilities have a nurse who specializes in breast examinations at nominal cost.)

BSE—when? Why should women perform BSE every month or so? Why not every two weeks or every two months?

A month is an interval long enough so that a woman's eyes and fingers can distinguish a change in the breast, but short enough so that they can "remember" what the breast was like before (harder to do when the interval is longer). Any significant change can be detected, diagnosed and treated as early as possible.

For the woman who menstruates (or still has functioning ovaries after a hysterectomy), this schedule means that the breasts are at the same stage of the hormonal cycle each time she examines them. In addition, it's easy to remember to do something once a month or so, because human lives tend to revolve around monthly cues (the first of the month, bills, menstrual period, and so on).

For women who menstruate, the best time to perform BSE is during the week after the menstrual period ends, when the hormones are at their lowest level and the breasts are least lumpy. Women past menopause, those who have had their ovaries removed—and women who currently are not ovulating because of pregnancy or breastfeeding—don't experience this significant hormonal rise and fall, so their breasts don't change so much from week to week. They still need to practice BSE monthly, but can pick any day that will jog their memory each month: the first of the month, perhaps, or the day they pay the mortgage.

Finding the right day can be trickier for the woman who has had a hysterectomy but still has functioning ovaries. She still experiences hormonal fluctuation, but may not be as aware of it as she was when she was menstruating. She needs to be alert to other cues, such as cyclic breast tenderness or lumpiness, or periodic weight gain, and to perform BSE when these symptoms of high hormonal levels are not present.

How to perform BSE. A complete self-examination includes *inspecting* the breasts, *palpating* them (feeling them with fingers and hands)—and *reporting* any changes to a health professional. It's easy to perform BSE. It takes practice to learn to do it with confidence, but there's nothing difficult about the procedure.

Inspection. The only things necessary for inspecting the breasts are eyes, a large mirror, good light, and a relaxed, unhurried approach. Inspection takes only a few minutes, but needs to be done very carefully, since it can offer evidence of a problem before there's a lump to feel.

What's a woman looking for? She's looking for what's normal for her—and seeing if there are any changes.

"But how do I know whether it's normal or a change if I've never examined my breasts carefully before?" asks Nancy. While it's helpful for a woman to have a health professional examine her breasts along with her the first time, pointing out what's normal for her, it's not worth waiting several months until a regular checkup before starting BSE. In most cases, the woman won't find anything alarming. If she does find something which worries her, a phoned description to the doctor usually brings reassurance.

Most women don't have perfectly-matched breasts. One breast is normally somewhat larger than the other and one may be higher on the chest than the other.

What is normal for one woman may represent change for another. Most women's nipples are *everted* (stick out from the breast), but others have nipples flat with the breast or even *inverted* (tucked into the areola). As long as a woman has had inverted nipples all along, that's normal for her; on the other hand, if this is a recent change, it needs to be investigated. Nipples come in all shapes and sizes and colors, and so do areolas—but the only thing that is worrisome is a change.

Some women have accessory breasts, additional bulges of breast tissue, sometimes with a small nipple, often located near or in the armpit; unless the bulges have changed, they are a normal variation. Veins may barely show through the skin or may be quite prominent, and still be absolutely normal. Aside from individual variations, most women develop prominent blood vessels during pregnancy and lactation.

What kind of changes should a woman look for, and why? She's looking for any dip or valley in the breast contour, or any change in how the nipple looks. Those delicate supporting fibers—Cooper's ligaments—that extend from the skin to the chest wall

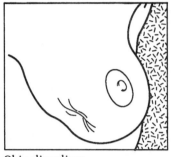

Skin dimpling

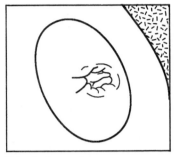

Nipple inversion

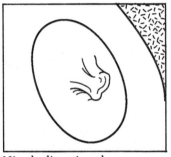

Nipple direction change

between the breast lobes, can be pulled out of position by a breast cancer, even before there's a lump to feel. This distortion, in turn, pulls on the skin, *retracting* or dimpling it, or on the nipple, inverting it or changing its direction.

She searches, too, for any swelling of the breast over a tumor, or for general puffiness caused by blocked lymph vessels. These show themselves as a change in the size of one breast or a bulge in contour;

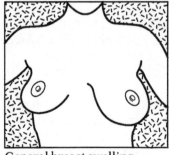

General breast swelling

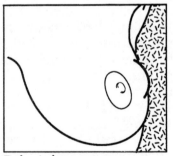

Bulge in breast contour

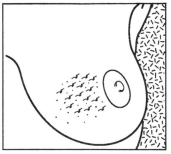

Large pores

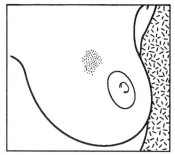

Reddened area

in addition, the stretched skin can become shiny or can thicken and develop large pores, rather like the peel of an orange. The skin can become reddened or discolored in one spot or a large area. The blood vessels can increase in number and prominence in one breast, as a tumor demands additional nutrition from the blood. A nipple can develop rashes or sores of different types.

Any of these

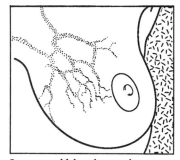

Increased blood vessels

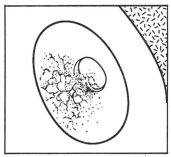

Nipple rash

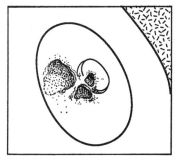

Nipple sore

changes can come from innocent breast processes—
and often does. The skin retraction turns out to be the
fold in a "stretch mark," after the breast has gained
and lost weight (after pregnancy, for instance). The
bulge may be a cyst, easily drained. With advancing
age, altered skin textures and elasticity can mimic
changes seen with breast cancer, such as skin dips and
dimpling. And so on. But *any* change like this needs to
be reported to a health professional.

To perform the inspection part of BSE, the
woman stands in front of the mirror and turns slowly

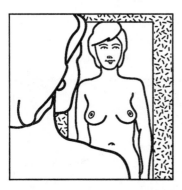 from side to side so that
the light reveals any dips
or bulges in the breast contour. (The woman with
decreased vision may find
a hand mirror more help-
ful.) She becomes
acquainted with her
breasts as she stands with
her arms at her sides. How
symmetrical are the
breasts? How does the skin
look? Any unusual patches of color? Are there stretch
marks, moles, or scars? Any thickened areas of skin
with large pores? Any puffy area or an obviously
swollen breast? How about the pattern of blood vessels under the skin?

There are better positions for accentuating any
breast swellings or dips. Thus, the woman raises her
arms, holding the elbows back and clasping her hands
behind the head; this position tightens the chest muscles, elevates the breasts, and stretches the skin. As
she pivots very slowly, she brings first one breast forward and then the other as she inspects them from

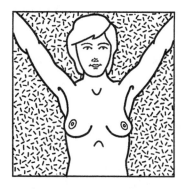 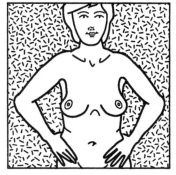

different angles. Then, hands pressing firmly on the hips, she turns again, looking for swelling, dimpling, puckering, or other change in contour.

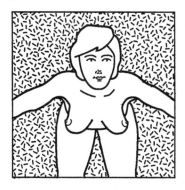

In his helpful booklet, *Breast Self-Examination*,* Dr. Albert R. Milan recommends a leaning-forward position as well. This involves bending at the hips so that the breasts hang straight down, while the woman supports her arms on the back of a chair or on her knees. This is a good position for checking the relative sizes of the breasts, and whether they hang symmetrically. A tumor may cause one breast to pull back toward the ribs.

In each position, the woman can lift a large and/ or pendulous breast with the opposite hand, so that

---

*Albert R. Milan, *Breast Self-Examination*, Workman Publishing, New York, 1980, pp. 80, 82-7.

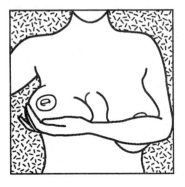

she can see the underside easily.

Nipples and areolas deserve special attention. It is important that the woman look not only at how symmetrical they are, which way the nipples point, whether they're inverted, flat or everted, but also at the skin itself. Are there any rashes, flaking skin, sores, or breaks in the skin?

Palpation. It's no mystery why women discover so many of their breast lumps accidentally while they're soaping in the shower. When they wash their breasts, women feel free to touch them, and slick, soapy breasts are easy to palpate. Unfortunately, most of the lumps found that way are relatively large, because it is not the most efficient way to explore all the breast tissue. The best palpation techniques combine that slippery, easy-to-feel sensation with more effective ways of finding *small* lumps.

"It all feels lumpy to me," moans Veronica. "How do I tell what's a 'real' lump?"

Some breast health programs provide breast models, with specific lumps as well as normal general lumpiness in them, so that women can educate their fingers to distinguish between the two, as well as to learn how to find progressively smaller lumps. Some breast models, including those with different degrees of background lumpiness to "match" the woman's own breasts, can be purchased and taken home after BSE training so that the woman can re-educate her fingers each month before examining her breasts.

Alternatively, a woman can make her own breast model, although it probably won't last as long as a purchased model. Dr. Milan suggests filling a sturdy plastic food bag not too full with warm gelatin, adding some partially cooked rice to simulate the feel of normal lumpiness, and allowing the gelatin to cool and firm.* If she adds a few "lumps" (a small gritty rock, a dried bean or pea, a grape, for example), the woman will be able to practice distinguishing lumps from general lumpiness. The practice lumps should be half an inch or smaller because that's the size of the breast lumps she wants to learn to detect.

The woman can jog her memory each month with the six P's of palpation: *placement* of the fingers; *pressures* of the fingers; *perimeter* (boundaries) of breast tissue to be examined; *position* of the breast; *pattern* for the fingers to follow in checking the breasts—and *practice.*

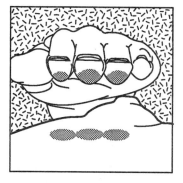

First, as she lies down with the practice breast model (if she has one) resting on the chest wall, and then with each breast, the woman *places* the flat area of the three middle fingers, from the last joint to the end of the finger, on the tissue to be examined. She uses the hand opposite the breast to be examined, and lays the fingers flat and parallel to the chest wall. The flats of the fingers are more sensitive than the fingertips, and the three-finger technique stabilizes the tissue so that a lump can't skitter away from probing fingers.

The MammaCare Method, one program of BSE training, recommends that the woman move the flats of the fingers in small, dime-sized circles, using three *pressures* at each spot. The light-pressure circle just

*Milan, p. 34

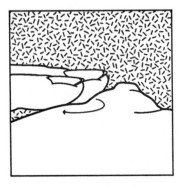

moves the skin without jostling the breast tissue underneath. The medium-pressure circle presses midway into the tissue, while the deep-pressure circle probes deeply, firmly into the breast, down to the ribs or to the point just short of discomfort.

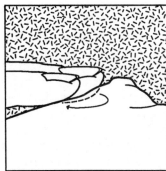

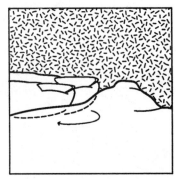

Breast lumps can appear at any depth in the breast, and this thoroughness gives a woman the best chance of finding anything that's there.

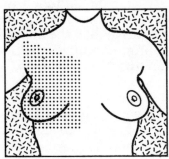

Shaded area is perimeter for BSE

The *perimeter* for BSE covers more area than just what fits into the bra. For each breast, it includes the area from the collarbone at the top to the braline at the bottom, and from the breastbone to an imaginary line drawn from the shoulder through the middle of the armpit, down the side to the braline.

The *position* for each breast supports and spreads the breast evenly so that all the tissue can be felt against the firm background of the chest wall. When most women stand, gravity pulls the breast tissue down so that it bulges at the bases; it's difficult to examine these bulges and harder to "trap" any lump. Lying down flat on the back is better, and is a position commonly recommended for BSE, but women with substantial breast tissue may find their breasts bulging to the sides.

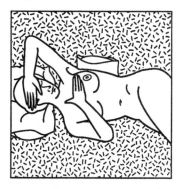

One way for a woman to avoid these bulges is to place a pillow under the shoulder of the side she plans to examine. MammaCare refines this technique: When a woman examines the outer half of her right breast, she turns onto her left side, bends her knees, and then lets her right shoulder fall back slightly until the nipple "floats" at the top of the mound of breast. A pillow behind her back makes the position comfortable. Like a languishing Victorian heroine, she rests the back of the right hand on her

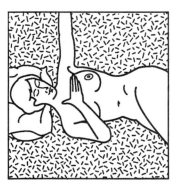

forehead. To examine the inner half of the right breast, from nipple line to breastbone, the woman pushes the pillow away and rolls onto her back. The arm is held straight out to the side.

After these preliminaries, which should take only a few seconds to recall after a woman has performed BSE a few times, she applies cornstarch or other powder, oil or lotion to the breast, so it's easier to feel. She can relubricate the breasts during the examination, if they lose their slippery feel.

There are three basic *patterns* for the fingers to follow in examining the breasts. Each has its advocates, and any one of them, done carefully and regularly, can be effective.

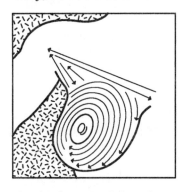

A traditional pattern, taught by the American Cancer Society in its BSE classes, involves examining the breasts in concentric rings. The fingers make their dime-sized circles beginning at the top of the breast, far from the nipple. After making circles at three pressures there, the fingers move clockwise one finger breadth and repeat the process. Once the fingers have completed their search all around the largest ring, they move inward toward the nipple to make another, smaller ring. Each ring gets smaller until the nipple is reached. It's very important to feel around and under the nipple (because

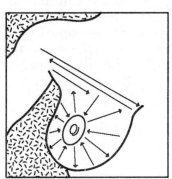

that's where many lumps get overlooked), and in the tail of breast tissue in the armpit.

A second pattern divides the breast into twelve sections like a clock, and draws imaginary lines from the nipple to each of the "numerals." The fingers move along each imaginary line making their small circles at different pressures: from "12" to the nipple, back from the nipple to "1," over to "2" and down the line to the nipple, and so on. Under the nipple and the armpit area are examined also.

The third pattern searches the breast tissue in

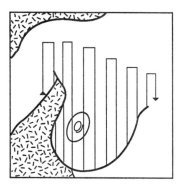

parallel lines, either horizontal or vertical. The MammaCare pattern uses vertical lines. Lying on her side, the woman moves her fingers in their small circles from the shoulder down an imaginary line through the armpit to the braline. At the end of that strip, the fingers move inward one finger breadth and start upward toward the collarbone. The fingers repeat up and down vertical strips until the fingers reach the nipple. They're held in place over the nipple as the woman rolls to her back, and then continue searching in parallel strips until they reach the breastbone.

Nipple discharges. Whichever pattern she uses to examine her breasts, the woman includes a check for

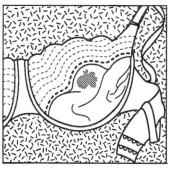

Nipple discharge on bra

any nipple discharge. Most doctors are more concerned with spontaneous nipple discharges—the stain inside the bra, for instance—than with those "milked" from the breast, but many recommend that a woman not only inspect her underwear but also attempt to express fluid from each breast.

Examining the Breasts **95**

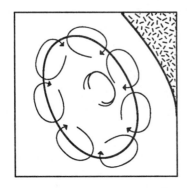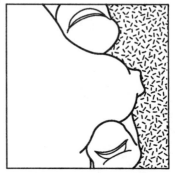

A good way to do this is to perform BSE small circles around the edge of the areola so that any fluid in the collecting reservoirs is massaged into the nipple area. Then the fingers, positioned on both sides of the nipple, press into the areola and come almost together under the nipple. The fingers are moved around the nipple a quarter circle and press again from that direction.

Even in women who aren't breastfeeding, a few drops of milky discharge from both breasts, or slight crusting at the tips of the nipples is common, and usually either normal or a sign of mild hormonal irregularity. Of more concern are copious milky discharges in a non-lactating woman, discharges from one breast, or any that are watery, sticky, yellow, pink, or obviously bloody (red to black color), or that have pus in them. Many of these come from benign breast processes, but they all need to be investigated.

What palpation findings mean. BSE isn't just a finger exercise, of course. Unless the sense of touch is closely connected to a questioning, concentrating, thinking *brain*, the examination is a waste of time. A woman is feeling for anything which is different from last month, and also for differences between the left and right breasts.

A woman has several kinds of tissue in her breasts, and the proportions change as she grows older. In the young woman, glandular, somewhat lumpy tissue, with a grainy feel (like partially cooked rice, cottage cheese, or pillow ticking) fills much of the central area of the breast.

Soft, fatty tissue tends to be found primarily at the periphery of the breast in premenopausal women, but gradually replaces the glandular tissue as women grow older. Fibrous tissue feels ridgy, rather like corrugations, or sometimes like a thick pancake; it appears in varying amounts in individual women at different ages.

As the woman palpates her breast, she's checking for any *dominant* three-dimensional lump, something that stands out from the surrounding area, or for new thickening—for anything that's new, different, a change. It can be quite small, the size of a kernel of popping corn, or much larger.

What if she finds "something"? First she checks the same area of the opposite breast to see if there's something similar there. If there is, the lumpiness or thickening is probably normal. For instance, many women have a "natural underwire," a thickened shelf at the base of each breast, or have thickening in the upper outer area of both breasts. These need to be checked carefully for any dominant lump, but usually represent normal breast tissue.

If she discovers something she thinks is new in one breast, the woman *reports it to her doctor or nurse. Right away.* In most cases, it will turn out to be a benign change, and she'll be reassured. In the rare case where the change means cancer, she enlists time as her friend by taking quick action.

As the member of the breast care team with the greatest familiarity with her own breasts, the woman needs to speak up, show, point, palpate, if necessary. This is not the time to sit back shyly and wait for the doctor or nurse to find the lump she has discovered (or to conclude that if the health professional doesn't locate it, no change exists).

Some women, especially those who form large cysts frequently, experience quite dramatic breast changes often. The doctor may want to give such a woman some additional instruction in BSE so that she doesn't have to visit the doctor *every* month. However, cysts are not always benign, and they need to be professionally evaluated (and probably drained) on a regular—if not an urgent—basis.

Not all women need to record their BSE findings from month to month, but it can be a big help for the woman with areas of general lumpiness. During her first exam, either with a health professional or by herself, the woman can "map" her breasts. Using a simple diagram (such as two large circles with axillary "tails," with smaller inner circles for areolas and nipples), she marks off any lumpy areas or thickenings. That way, from month to month she doesn't become alarmed about the same findings.

The professional breast exam

The second component of a complete breast health program is the professional breast examination. Whether these exams are performed by a doctor or nurse, they need to be thorough and scheduled on a regular basis. Preferably, the same person performs the examination each time, and gains some familiarity with the woman's breasts.

How can a woman tell if her professional breast exam is reasonably thorough? It does not need to be lengthy, but it must contain *at least* the following elements: a breast history of risk factors and past problems, taken during the first visit; questioning about any current breast concerns; visual inspection under good light, with the woman standing or sitting with arms both down and raised; careful palpation of all the breast tissue—including that in the armpits, along the collarbones, and beneath the nipples— while a woman lies down with arms behind her head. (There are several effective patterns and styles for palpation. By following the same routine through examination of numerous women, the health professional becomes familiar with the variations in the normal breast so that any deviation is more obvious.)

The examination should be carried out with respect for the woman's dignity and modesty. If the professional breast exam does not meet these minimum standards of thoroughness and concern for the patient, the woman needs to speak up or change health professionals.

Many doctors or nurses perform much more thorough breast exams. Some use additional patient positions for visual inspection and/or palaption. Many teach as they examine the breasts. Some routinely try to extract any nipple discharge with a special suction device, and send any cells obtained for examination under a microscope; how effective this is as a general screening procedure is still in question.

How often should professional breast exams be done? A common-sense schedule for women under 40 without breast complaints or special risk factors calls for a breast exam at least every two to three years, perhaps conveniently combined with the gynecological check-up and Pap smear. The woman over 40 needs an annual breast exam. If a woman needs more frequent breast checks, because of substantial breast cancer risk factors, continuing breast problems (such as recurrent cysts), or increasing age, the health professional and the woman can discuss when and how often exams should occur. Of course, if a woman finds breast changes during BSE, she notifies her doctor or nurse.

With her own educated fingers, eyes, and brain, and those of a knowledgeable, thorough health professional, a woman has two-thirds of the best breast health program she can get.

Picturing the Breast: Mammograms and Such

When Dr. Virginia Griswold, radiologist, first told the surgeons at her hospital what she expected of them, they were dumbfounded.

"Surgeons trust their fingers and what they can *feel*. But here was I, the new radiologist, reading mammograms and recommending breast biopsies on the basis of something that could be seen on an X-ray but not felt. They'd say, 'You want me to do a biopsy because of some tiny white specks on a film? You're kidding, aren't you?'

"I won't say we almost came to blows, but there was a *lot* of conflict at first. Now most of them have become true believers!"

Mammography

By the time a cancerous lump can be felt in the breast, it usually contains more than a billion cells. It has been growing for several years, doubling from one cell to two, from two cells to four and, in time, from one billion cells to two billion.

Originally, doctors used mammograms—the special X-rays which show the internal structures of the breast—primarily to confirm a lump they could feel. During the 1960's, however, mammography matured into a screening technique for large groups of women without disease symptoms. As radiologists saw more and more breast films, they noticed that at times certain features in a mammogram (particularly calcium deposits) which often accompanied cancerous lumps could be seen even when there was no lump to be seen or felt. Could these changes, they wondered, be early signs of cancer?

Joining forces with surgeons and pathologists, the radiologists discovered that while these X-ray changes most often signaled benign breast processes, in many cases they revealed cancer or carcinoma in situ. (Mammography only *detects* signs that *might* be cancer; *diagnosis* requires a biopsy or other test.)

The radiologists were jubilant. When cancer is detected and diagnosed this early, before there is a lump to palpate, it is almost always curable, often with minimal treatment.

What mammography shows. What clues is the radiologist searching for on a mammogram? Dr. Frederick Margolin, chief radiologist at Children's Hospital of San Francisco, summarizes: "If this is a woman's first mammogram, and I don't have anything to compare it to, I look for several things.

"I check for *symmetry*: In most women, the right breast isn't too different from the left. I check the amount and kind of tissue. Are there any abnormal-appearing *lumps or localized densities*? What about the *architecture of the breast*? (The lacy network of fibers in the breast can be distorted by a cancer even before we can see the cancer itself.) I observe the *skin* for thickening or irregularity. I check the *axilla* (armpit) for anything unusual.

"Finally, I use a magnifying glass to see if there are any *clusters of calcifications*. That's probably our most helpful early sign that there might be a cancer developing—or an area of duct carcinoma in situ.

"Of course, if I have an earlier mammogram for comparison, I look for any *changes* that have occurred since the last examination."

Obviously, radiologists are curious about any large "lump" appearing on a mammogram. Each lump has characteristics—like shape, regularity of outline, density and the presence or absence of a "halo" (or lighter area) around it—which are clues to whether it is benign or cancerous. But radiologists are especially interested in the subtle changes that can't be seen or felt during physical examination of the breast: lumps too small to palpate, calcifications (also called microcalcifications), and architectural distortions.

It is sometimes difficult to tell if abnormalities seen in a mammogram mean benign disease or cancer. Calcifications, for instance, those tiny white specks of calcium salts left as cellular debris, can appear in a cluster with ductal cancer—or as benign changes after inflammation or injury of the breast, or when the ducts become plugged with debris which can calcify. Radiologists look at the size and shape of each individual speck, and at the number and pattern of calcifications, for clues as to whether the cluster is benign or cancerous. A small number of round calcifications is less worrisome than a large number of long, branching calcifications.

Similarly, architectural distortions sometimes mean cancer, but often don't. Radiologists look with special care at stellate (star-shaped) gatherings of fibers; an unseen cancer can be pulling the fibers into this unusual conformation.

If there's something questionable on the mammogram, the radiologist may recommend either immediate biopsy or a follow-up mammogram in a few months, depending on *how* suspicious the finding is. No radiologist wants to put a woman through the anxiety, discomfort, and expense of a biopsy without sufficient reason; on the other hand, no radiologist —or patient—wants to miss a cancer if it's there.

Dr. Margolin considers mammography an art rather than an exact science. Some findings on a mammogram are clear-cut. Others require a judgment call, based on a radiologist's training and experience. We depend on the radiologist's expertise, sensitivity, and even hunches, and it makes sense to ask questions: Does the radiologist deal with mammograms every day or, at least, quite often? Any special training in mammography?

Mammography complements physical

examination. Some abnormalities show up on one, some on the other, and some on both. If there's a palpable lump which doesn't appear on the mammogram, most radiologists would defer to a surgeon's judgment about whether it needs aspiration or biopsy.

Machines and techniques. What about the machines? Both mammography and Xeromammography (or Xeroradiography, pronounced "Zero. . .") use X-rays to visualize the breast. The differences between the two lie in the recording devices and the final product. A mammogram is an X-ray *film*, with breast structures in black and white, like a large photographic negative. In contrast, a Xeromammogram (or Xeroradiograph) uses electrostatic energy to produce a blue and white picture on *paper*; the technique was developed by the Xerox Corporation—hence the name.

The two techniques provide pictures of comparable quality. Some radiologists prefer one technique over the other, largely because their training and experience have made them more familiar with that one.

Getting a mammogram. What happens when a woman is scheduled for a mammogram?

Each X-ray department issues its own preliminary instructions. Most recommend that the woman wear a blouse or other easily removable clothing above the waist. Deodorant, perfume, powder, and even poorly rinsed soap on the breast and armpit area can cause misleading findings on the mammogram, and should be washed off before the examination. The woman may be asked to complete a form detailing her breast and reproductive history, risk factors, and any breast symptoms. If there is any possibility that the woman is pregnant, mammography is postponed if possible; if the mammogram is urgent, the woman will need special protection (usually a lead apron below the breasts).

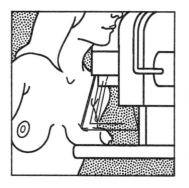

For the exam, a technician flattens the entire breast between two hard plastic layers, appropriately called a *compressor*. (There are other kinds of breast-compressing devices, but this is the most common type.) To produce the picture, the X-rays pass through an opening in the machine and then through the breast, exposing the film beneath.

Ordinarily, the technician takes two or three pictures of each breast from different angles, repositioning machine, breast, and the woman's arms for each image. For each mammogram, the technician steps away from the machine, tells the woman to stop breathing for a few seconds, and takes the picture. The technician develops the films, and the radiologist checks them to be sure the quality is adequate and that no additional views are needed before the woman leaves. Later, the radiologist's written report is sent to the woman's doctor.

Sometimes, the radiologist wants *magnification views* of a questionable area. These pictures enlarge a small area one-and-a-half to two times, and show it in much greater detail. This may either calm the radiologists's suspicions or confirm them. From the patient's point of view, the process is the same, except that the breast is positioned with special care so that the questionable area is at the center of the picture.

In case of a suspicious breast discharge or other nipple/areola irregularity, the doctor may want more detail of that area than the routine mammogram captures, and may arrange for a *duct X-ray*. For this, the radiologist gently enlarges one (or more) of the pores at the end of the nipple and carefully injects a small amount of special fluid until the woman experiences a sensation of fullness. This fluid shows up clearly on the X-ray to outline the suspect duct(s). This procedure is seldom necessary, however, and is used only rarely.

Why don't more women get mammograms? The technique is simple and life-saving. Why do so many women hesitate?

1. "I'm scared of what they'll find." It's a normal reaction to be afraid of the unknown. However, most screening mammograms show normal breasts, without a hint of cancer—and are reassuring. In the unlikely case of cancer, the scary part is *not* finding it early.

Of course, mammography doesn't change what's happening inside the breast; it simply detects it. If there is anything suspicious going on inside there, I, for one, want to find it as early as possible so that it can be cured with the least possible disruption in my life. That's what regular screening mammograms offer.

2. "It hurts." When Ann Landers printed a letter from "N.Y. Victim" complaining about pain from a mammogram, she was inundated with letters. Women called for revenge on the "male [who] invented that diabolical machine."

Yes, it can be uncomfortable—but it should *not* be painful and should not cause bruising. That's a lesson I've had to learn the hard way, as a veteran of frequent mammograms (as follow-up for calcifications), which usually include repeat and magnification views. (Once, after a painful session with an over-zealous student technician, I discovered that one large and prominent cyst had disappeared, presumably popped by a very forceful compression!)

It's much more comfortable for women who menstruate to have mammograms taken during the first half of the menstrual cycle, when the breasts are softer and less likely to be tender; the pictures may be a little clearer, too, with the breasts at relative rest. (I have friends who swear by eliminating caffeine from the diet for two weeks before mammography: coffee, tea, cola, and chocolate. Some X-ray departments recommend this in their preliminary instructions.)

And I've learned that the technician makes a big difference, and that I can speak up, if necessary. The breasts do need to be flattened somewhat for a clear picture with the newer "low-dose" techniques, which deliver smaller amounts of radiation than older processes. However, the primary elements of the "low-dose" technology are the sensitivity of the film and the improved focusing of the X-rays themselves, rather that the compression of the breast.

Squeezing the breasts more to get good pictures of difficult-to-visualize breasts is like shouting at a person with impaired hearing: It doesn't work. Accurate films can be taken with *reasonable* compression. Many experienced technicians compress the breasts to the point of discomfort, then release the pressure a tiny bit. Also, the compression lasts only a few seconds.

"Sure, it's uncomfortable," agrees Dr. Griswold, "but any woman who would refuse to have mammograms for that reason needs to do a lot more thinking."

Dr. Griswold should know. As a radiologist, she reads mammograms all the time. As a woman, she undergoes periodic mammography. And as a daughter, she saw her mother's early and minimal cancer detected by mammography, long before there was a lump to feel.

3. *"Is it safe?"* There is *no* evidence that mammography has ever induced a breast cancer, even with older, higher-dose techniques.

Dr. Margolin believes that, "Like everything else, it's a risk-benefit ratio. We know that large doses of radiation, like at Hiroshima (100 rads or more in a single exposure) are associated with increased numbers of breast cancers 15 years or more down the road. This is especially true if the radiation was received by a very young woman, with rapidly growing tissue that is more susceptible to radiation damage.

"But mammography delivers 1000 times less radiation than that, and many experts believe such tiny doses are harmless. With newer mammogram machines, it is estimated that the risk of developing a breast cancer from the radiation exposure of a mammogram is equivalent to the lung cancer risk of smoking half of one cigarette. Even if such a cancer did develop after 10-20 years, it would most probably be detected by the mammogram while it was early and curable.

"We have the proven benefit of early detection of breast cancer when it's curable versus a theoretical risk. *It's no contest!"*

For our maximum safety, what questions do we need to ask? Is this a *dedicated* mammography unit, one intended and used only for mammography? Is this *low-dose* radiation equipment? (The total dose of radiation for all views of each breast should be one rad or less.) How old is this equipment? (Machines less than five years old are preferred, because they incorporate the safest new technology and have fewer chances of equipment malfunction.) Does the technician have special training in mammography?

4. *"It's expensive."* Some insurance policies and most health maintenance organizations pay all or part of the costs of mammography. In addition, prices

vary considerably from facility to facility. In my community, there's a mobile van which provides screening mammograms (read by a radiologist simply as "normal," "abnormal," or "questionable"), at about one-quarter the cost of those done in an office or hospital with direct radiologist supervision. Or we might decide to put aside a few dollars each month to pay for periodic mammograms.

False-positives and false-negatives. Mammography is an effective tool for detecting cancer—but it is not perfect. On the average, the mammogram will find nine out of 10 breast cancers. It is more accurate in some women than in others. Breasts containing moderately large amounts of fat are ideal for mammography, as even the smallest abnormality is easily detected. On the other end of the spectrum is the very dense breast with little or no fat. As the fat acts as a background on which the silhouette of breast structures is portrayed, its absence makes the mammogram more difficult to interpret.

Viewing the mammograms of a woman with very dense breasts is like looking through a thick fog. Density comes from normal working breast tissue in young women, from individual variations in the numbers and arrangement of ducts and glands, and from benign breast changes, such as cysts and overgrown fibrous tissue.

Breast changes *may* show up distinctly in even the most dense breasts. However, radiologists are much less confident that they will see a lump, thickening or change in the breast architecture of dense breasts, although calcifications sometimes show up quite clearly.

If our breasts are especially dense, we need to know about it. "Very dense breasts," as mentioned on a mammography report, refers to a visual finding, but it also means that we must rely more on our fingers and eyes and on our doctor's breast examinations—and less on mammograms—than we would otherwise. The doctor may recommend ultrasound or another imaging technique, or a diagnostic test if there's a question about a specific area. As the years pass, the dense breast tissue is replaced by fatty tissue, which makes the breasts easier to visualize on mammograms.

Because of their shape, with most of the breast tissue right at the chest wall, very small breasts can be a challenge to compress and mammograph accurately. Dr. Margolin claims, however, that even quite small as well as very large breasts can usually be examined adequately with careful technique.

Since about one of every ten breast cancers will not be found by X-ray, mammography has approximately a 10% *false negative* rate even when performed and interpreted very carefully. This reinforces the importance of BSE and professional physical examination of the breasts.

False positive results occur too. The mammogram may show worrisome calcifications which are not associated with a cancer, a lump which may be a benign tumor, or changes due to old inflammation or injury. As all of these may be suspicious findings to the radiologist, biopsy may be suggested. Two out of three times, when a mammogram prompts a biopsy, no cancer or duct carcinoma in situ is found.

Mammograms—when? How often should women have mammograms? Baseline mammography between ages 35 and 40 gives the radiologist comparison films for later years when cancerous changes would be more likely to occur. (Before age 35, breast tissue tends to be too dense to visualize well, and is particularly sensitive to the effects of radiation.)

Current American Cancer Society guidelines call for mammography every one to two years between ages 40 and 50, depending on a woman's risk factors and symptoms, and every year after that. Both Dr. Margolin and Dr. Griswold believe that these guidelines will be reversed eventually, to recommend mammograms yearly between ages 40 and 50, and every two years after that. Their rationale is that breast cancers which appear before menopause tend to grow faster than those which occur later in life; thus, surveillance every two years after age 50 should be adequate to detect cancerous changes at an early, curable stage.

Periodic mammograms are appropriate to follow up certain X-ray findings (when the appearance is not sufficiently suspicious for an immediate biopsy), or to check something newly discovered during physical examination. The frequency of such follow-up examinations varies with what's being evaluated, but is seldom more often than every four to six months.

Other imaging techniques

Mammography is currently the workhorse of breast-imaging techniques. Nothing approaches it for all-around accuracy, both for screening breasts without symptoms and for imaging breasts where a problem is suspected.

But it's not a perfect technique, and some day another procedure—either one already available or one not yet imagined—may challenge mammography. Currently, other processes are used in tandem with mammography and/or in a few specific situations where they are better. None has demonstrated the ability of mammography to detect duct carcinoma in situ and early invasive breast cancer, however.

Ultrasound projects high-frequency sound waves into the breast. The sound waves bounce off different kinds of tissue in characteristic ways. A computer then reads the pattern of echoes and produces a visual representation of the breast.

The technique works best in showing whether a particular mass is solid or fluid-filled, especially in very dense breasts. It also shows the area close to the chest wall, an area often difficult to image with mammography. It may be safer than mammography early in pregnancy, or for women under 30 if a suspicious lump is found by palpation. However, ultrasound doesn't show calcifications, changes in breast architecture or some small lumps that mammography would detect, and is thus at a disadvantage in finding in situ carcinoma or very early invasive breast cancer.

For an ultrasound examination using an automated water path scanner, the woman lies on her stomach and immerses her breasts in a tank of warm water; alternatively, she positions the breasts in a special water cushion. Another technique, which many radiologists prefer, is to use a hand-held instrument placed directly on the breast.

Ultrasound examination is a painless procedure which takes 15 to 30 minutes.

Thermography and other heat-sensing techniques capitalize on the fact that the body radiates, or throws off, heat—more of it in areas with greater blood flow. In theory, if a rapidly-growing tumor demands more nutrition from an increased blood supply, a detectable "hot spot" may develop. Each technique uses a different kind of material (heat-sensitive crystals, for instance, or a probe) to sense temperature changes.

Heat-sensing processes show cancers that are fairly large and/or near the surface of the breast which produce marked temperature changes at skin level. They do not detect deep tumors well, and don't give the information about in situ carcinoma or early signs of cancer that mammography can.

Before a thermogram, the woman sits in a cool room until her skin temperature lowers. Then her breasts are placed against the sensitive material, which registers any temperature variations, often with different colors.

In *diaphanography* (transillumination), light shining through the breast shows the breast interior. A fiberoptic device (a tube containing special light-sending fibers) directs infrared light through the breast; the transmitted light is then photographed with infrared film. To the trained examiner, healthy breast tissue, a cyst, a benign tumor, or a cancerous tumor each has a characteristic color and appearance.

Diaphanography does not show calcifications or changes in breast architecture. It cannot accurately distinguish cancer from mastitis or bleeding.

There is no known risk from diaphanography.

Computed tomography (CT) can find some cancers in small, very dense breasts, but it is a poor screening technique because it uses relatively large doses of X-rays, requires an injection into the vein, and is quite expensive. *Magnetic resonance imaging* (MRI; it used to be called nuclear magnetic resonance or NMR) uses an interaction of magnetism and radiowaves to image the breast structures. It appears to be safe, though expensive, but has not yet proven it can detect small tumors or distinguish malignant tumors from benign ones.

A new imaging technique still being researched uses *monoclonal antibodies*: perfect, laboratory-produced copies (clones) of cancer antibodies. Experimenters add a dye or other marker to these antibodies, inject them into the body where they find and cling to any cancer cells, and then use special X-rays to take pictures. This works best as a follow-up procedure for a woman who has undergone treatment for breast cancer; her own antibodies to her particular cancer are cloned. It is *not* a general screening technique. As the test moves out of the experimental stage, it should become less expensive and more readily available.

Someday, we'll learn how to prevent breast cancer. Until that day, we rely on the earliest possible detection, diagnosis, and treatment of any breast cancer that does occur. We want a test that detects any and every breast cancer in any woman dependably, accurately, early, safely, and inexpensively.

Right now, mammography is the best we have—but maybe tomorrow...?

Diagnosing Breast Changes

It's hard to improve on fingers and eyes and mammograms to *detect* breast changes, to find the signs and symptoms which suggest that a problem exists. But for *diagnosis*—which says conclusively what those signs and symptoms *mean*—we need cells or tissue from the breast for examination under a microscope. Cells come from needle aspiration of the breast or a nipple discharge; tissue, which is made up of groups of similar cells, comes from breast biopsy.

What breast changes need diagnosis? (1) A dominant palpable lump (as opposed to general lumpiness), which persists throughout the menstrual cycle or which appears in a postmenopausal woman. (2) Tissue which appears markedly abnormal on mammography—a lump that can't be palpated, particular kinds of clustered calcifications, or certain architectural distortions. (3) Suspicious nipple discharges.

Diagnostic procedures, including needle aspirations, biopsies (both conventional and by needle localization), and cytologic examinations, are done to answer the question, "Does this breast change mean cancer?" Usually the answer is "No, it doesn't."

Based on the evidence of a thorough breast examination (and often a mammogram), the surgeon often can predict before the procedure what will be found. But there's no way of *knowing* until the report comes back, and often the educated guess before the procedure turns out to be wrong—which is why diagnostic examinations are necessary. According to *The Breast Cancer Digest*, "approximately 30 percent of all lesions thought to be cancer are not, and 15 percent of those believed benign turn out to be malignant."*

The most important part of any diagnostic procedure is obtaining the right tissue or cells. If there are cancer cells in a suspicious area, they may be

---

*National Cancer Institute, *The Breast Cancer Digest*, second edition, Besthesda, Maryland, 1984, p. 41.

gathered in one tiny spot. Thus, a biopsy which removes 95% of the problem area, but leaves the 5% where the cancer cells happen to be, will appear negative for cancer. This means that any diagnostic procedure must be performed as carefully and thoroughly as possible.

Needle aspiration

When is it done? When the doctor suspects that a breast lump is a fluid-filled cyst, fine needle aspiration (FNA) is a quick, simple, relatively inexpensive test that often solves the problem as well as diagnoses it. Aspiration is also used sometimes to withdraw a few cells from a solid lump or thickened area.

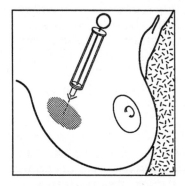 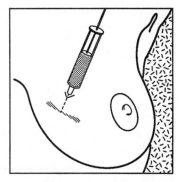

How is it done? In the office, the surgeon (or gynecologist or family doctor, perhaps) swabs the area with an antiseptic solution, inserts a thin hypodermic needle into the lump, and tries to aspirate, or withdraw, any fluid. Some doctors inject a local anesthetic first to numb the area. (My surgeon believes that injecting the anesthetic hurts as much as the insertion of the aspiration needle, so he doesn't use one.)

Cyst fluid normally comes in a wide range of colors, but shouldn't have blood in it. If the fluid looks suspicious and/or the lump doesn't collapse, the fluid is sent to the *cytology* laboratory to be checked under the microscope for any cancer cells. (This type of laboratory, where *cells* are examined, investigates nipple discharges as well as cells from needle aspirations.) Results are available within a few days.

How trustworthy are the results? If the lump collapses after fluid is aspirated and does not return, the diagnosis is almost certainly a benign cyst. If the report on cells is negative for cancer cells, it confirms the diagnosis. The area should still be checked monthly during BSE by the woman and periodically by the doctor. Sometimes cysts tend to refill with fluid even when they are benign. One or two additional aspirations of a cyst may be done before resorting to a surgical biopsy.

If the cells show cancer (are *positive* for cancer), the report can be trusted. The problem comes when the "cyst" does not collapse or is obviously a solid lump, and the report shows no cancer cells. *This negative report is not a sufficient diagnosis*; biopsy is advisable.

As Dr. Michael Lagios, pathologist at Children's Hospital of San Francisco, states about the "cyst" that doesn't collapse after aspiration, "It should be noted that a negative fine needle aspiration and a negative mammogram. . .in no way precludes carcinoma from being present. Too often women are reassured that because a fine needle aspiration is negative and a mammogram is negative that their lump is benign. Only months later when the lump actually grows in size and is finally biopsied is it apparent that they had an invasive carcinoma all along."

Sometimes, a surgeon uses a "wide needle," a larger-bore needle with a cutting edge, to remove a small piece of tissue under local anesthetic. Doctors may call this a needle biopsy, which should not be confused with a needle localization biopsy (see p. 126), a different procedure altogether. Or the surgeon may insert a thin needle several times in different directions into a solid lump to gather cells from different locations in the lump. These procedures are most appropriate when there is strong evidence that a lump or thickened area is cancerous and the surgeon wants confirmation before major breast surgery, without subjecting the patient to a biopsy also. Again, however, while a positive result can be trusted, a negative one is inconclusive.

Does an aspiration hurt? As a veteran of several aspirations, I've found it minimally uncomfortable when a large, obvious cyst was drained (like the discomfort of getting a blood test from a skilled technician, for instance). It is more painful—but briefly so—when the lump turns out to be a solid one, after several tries at aspiration. Sometimes there's an ache and/or a bruise for a few days, sometimes not.

Needle aspirations are popular with doctors and patients alike. They provide diagnosis and treatment simultaneously for cysts, one of the most common benign breast changes. Aspiration costs a small fraction of what a biopsy costs, takes a few minutes or less, and can be done on the spur of the moment, so that there's no anxious waiting for a biopsy. There's no scar on the breast, and no scar tissue inside the breast to make future examinations and mammograms more difficult to interpret. If it's used appropriately—for the diagnosis of fluid-filled lumps—it's the technique of choice.

Conventional surgical biopsy

When is it done? A conventional surgical biopsy is a diagnostic technique for a persistent, palpable, dominant, solid breast lump or thickened area or for a recurrent cyst.

How is it done? The lump or other suspicious area is removed, either all or in part. An *excisional biopsy* excises, or cuts out, the whole lump, often with a border of surrounding tissue; an *incisional biopsy* incises, or cuts into the suspicious area and removes part of it.

If the lump in an otherwise-healthy woman can be felt easily, is smaller that an inch or so in diameter, and is probably benign, the biopsy can be done under local anesthetic in a minor surgery room at the surgeon's office or as an outpatient procedure in the hospital. (Surgeons rely on their experienced fingers and on mammograms to tell them which lumps are *probably* benign.)

Surgeon or patient may prefer that she be admitted to the hospital, perhaps as a "same day surgery" patient who arrives in the morning before the biopsy and leaves the same afternoon or evening. This patient can be put to sleep with a general anesthetic if that's desirable (for removal of a lump deep within the breast, for example).

Wherever the biopsy is performed, the surgeon first explains the procedure and its risks to the woman and she signs a surgical consent, authorizing the removal of a piece of tissue from the breast. The consent may specify also that the doctor can sample tissue from the armpit area.

When I underwent my first biopsy several years ago, when women routinely were put to sleep for the procedure, I signed a consent giving the surgeon carte blanche: I didn't know whether I'd wake up to a small bandage or a missing breast. Now, unless there's a firm diagnosis of cancer before the biopsy—from a needle aspiration, perhaps—surgeons tend to perform the biopsy one day; then, if the final pathology report confirms breast cancer, the woman is given some additional days to review alternatives before any major breast surgery is done. This time separation of biopsy from definitive surgery is what makes a *two-step procedure*.

Waiting a few days before any definitive surgery does not seem to make any difference in the outcome if the diagnosis is breast cancer. It prevents unnecessary surgeries based on an inaccurate diagnosis from the preliminary pathology report, and it means that women don't have to wonder whether they'll come out of a biopsy with a tiny scar or a missing breast.

For the biopsy itself, the breast and surrounding area are swabbed generously and repeatedly with antiseptic solution and are draped so that only the operative area shows. The surgeon may draw the proposed incision line and lump location with a marking pen. The area is numbed with injections of a local anesthetic, or the woman is put to sleep with a general anesthetic. (Some surgeons give the woman a relaxing premedication.)

The surgeon cuts the skin and underlying tissue to reveal the lump, and removes the whole thing if it's reasonably small. (Most benign lumps push aside other breast tissue; when the lump is taken out, the other tissue springs back to fill any cavity, although the process may take time.)

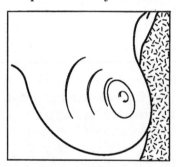

Natural curve of breast

Most surgeons try to follow the curve of the areola or the natural curve of the breast when making an incision, because the scar from such a cut is less noticeable when it heals. Rarely, a straight incision like a wheel spoke is necessary. It's worth asking before the biopsy what kind of incision the surgeon plans.

What's all this like for the woman lying awake on the operating table? She feels sensations of pressure and tugging; if she feels any pain, more local anesthetic is necessary. She hears the unfamiliar sounds of scalpel and scissors and the faint hiss of the electric cauterizing wand as it stops bleeding from tiny blood vessels. It's usually difficult to see much, even if the woman is so inclined. Some surgeons are talkative, some silent.

The surgeon often sends the specimen for an immediate *frozen section* while the woman is still in the operating room. The pathologist quick-freezes a piece of the specimen, slices it thinly, stains it, and examines it under the microscope. This prompt report, about 98% accurate, can tell the surgeon if more tissue needs to be removed. (The pathologist bases the final report, available in a few days, on a *permanent section* of tissue, painstakingly prepared in a process that takes about 24 hours.)

The surgeon stitches together the underlying tissues of the breast with sutures which don't need to be removed. The skin is closed with special tape strips or nonabsorbable sutures. (Tape strips fall off or are removed by the woman in about two weeks, and skin sutures are taken out by the surgeon in about a week.) The area is bandaged, and the woman goes home if the biopsy was performed under local anesthetic, or to the recovery room, if a general anesthetic was used. Time elapsed is usually well under an hour, with only a portion of that time spent on actual cutting and stitching.

How trustworthy are the results? If the suspicious area is removed completely, and the slides are prepared and interpreted by an experienced pathologist, the final report should be very reliable. For an area which is difficult to classify for any reason, the pathologist can send slides to consulting pathologists for their opinions.

Does it hurt? Injecting local anesthetic into the breast smarts for a few seconds. The surgery itself can be uncomfortable because of the strange sensations—

but shouldn't be painful unless it's time to ask for more local anesthetic. Afterwards, there is usually some pain the day of surgery, relieved by prescription pain pills. By the next day or so, discomfort ordinarily diminishes to occasional soreness, a feeling of tightness as the breast swells after surgery, and often some itching. The amount of discomfort depends on a woman's individual pain threshold and on the extent and type of surgical procedure.

Both swelling and bruising can be dramatic—but short-lived. A bra with firm support and/or a pillow to stabilize the breast at night can be comforting. Swelling, bruising, and tape strips or stitches vanish within two weeks or so; given some time, most scars become almost invisible. Complications from a breast biopsy are rare: infection or bleeding into the biopsy cavity.

The surgeon gives directions about how soon to remove the bandage, bathe, and resume normal—and more strenuous—activities. Most women can resume most normal occupations within a day or two.

Jogging or other activities which jar the breast repeatedly (or in which the arm is raised above shoulder level) should be avoided for two weeks or more, as the surgeon advises, and a firm supporting bra should be worn until the breast is fully healed. The avid exerciser can switch temporarily to activity which jolts the breast less (biking rather than jogging, for instance), and can consult the doctor about the earliest *safe* return to habitual exercise routines.

Needle localization biopsy

When is it done? When the breast abnormality is a mammographic finding rather that a palpable lump, the surgeon turns to the radiologist for help in "localizing" the suspicious area. This procedure can be done for a lump too small or deep to feel, a cluster of calcifications, or an architectural distortion in a breast.

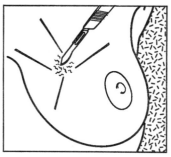
Needle localization

How is it done? The idea behind a needle localization biopsy is that the radiologist will mark the suspicious area of the breast with one or more needles (and often some dye), so that the surgeon can find the area and excise it.

Before the biopsy, the woman goes to the X-ray department for the localization part of the procedure. Radiologists have individual preferences. Some take an initial set of mammograms with a grid superimposed on them, and use the grid as a guide for needle placement. Others study mammogram views taken from different angles, and plot where the needle(s) will go.

After applying antiseptic solution and perhaps injecting some local anesthetic into the skin, the radiologist places one or more needles into the suspicious area. Some use a needle with a curved end or a small barb so that it stays where it's put; others use a straight needle, or one with fine wire threaded through it, which is left in for the biopsy after the needle is removed. Some radiologists place one needle, some more.

After the correct needle placement is confirmed by another mammogram, many radiologists inject a small amount of harmless blue dye to delineate the area further. The dye may sting for a short while. A bandage covers the area as the woman goes to the operating room for a biopsy.

Surgeons are more likely to choose a hospital operating room and a general anesthetic for this

Diagnosing Breast Changes   **127**

procedure than they are for a conventional biopsy, though many needle localization biopsies are performed under local anesthetic. Finding the "X marks the spot" area with a scalpel can be tedious and time-consuming, even with needle(s) and dye as guides.

As with a conventional biopsy, there are the routine trappings of a surgery: a consent form; the swabbing and draping of the breast; the injection of anesthetic, either local or general; and the closure of the biopsy wound.

What happens to the specimen after biopsy is different, however. Since the abnormality was apparent only on the mammogram, the specimen of tissue is X-rayed (*specimen radiographed*) to be sure that the correct area—and all of it—was excised. For instance, if microcalcifications were the abnormality, the specimen radiograph is compared to the mammogram taken before the biopsy to check that all the microcalcifications seen earlier are present in the excised tissue, with an area of normal tissue around them. Also, the pathologist, after slicing the tissue, may use X-rays again, especially with tissue slices at the edges of the specimen, to be sure that all the calcifications are well-contained within the specimen, with none right at the edges.

How trustworthy are the results? As long as the suspicious area is completely removed, the biopsy report should be reliable. Dr. Lagios cautions that needle localization biopsies are expensive and more difficult to perform correctly than conventional biopsies—so women need to ask questions beforehand: How familiar are the surgeon, radiologist, and pathologist with needle localization biopsies? (Since the procedure is a relatively new one, many physicians are not experienced in performing it.) Do they perform needle localization biopsies often? What localization technique does the radiologist use? Is the specimen routinely checked with specimen radiography? Are all the members of the team Board Certified in their specialities?

Dr. Lagios says, "A false negative biopsy, that is, one which is stated to not contain carcinoma where the lesion has not been sampled because of improper localization technique by the radiology department or inadequate preparation by the pathology department can be very devastating."

Does a needle localization biopsy hurt? Discomfort is comparable to that with a conventional biopsy, and so are swelling, bruising, and post-biopsy care.

Feelings about a biopsy

There's no such thing as "just a biopsy." It's anything but routine for the woman who undergoes one.

In her short article, "No Biopsy Is Routine,"* LeeAn Lowe writes: "Thousands have biopsies every year. If you are one of those people, you know the utter helplessness of lying on the operating table. You know the fear of being cut, and you know the terrible, gnawing dread that they might find what they're looking for."

She found herself angry—outraged—after the biopsy, and her feelings aren't unusual. She was "hardly pleased about being cut up in order to find out I'm perfectly healthy. . ." (And most women undergoing biopsies have the same experience of finding that they're perfectly healthy: about three-quarters of those with conventional biopsies, and about two-thirds of those with needle localization biopsies.)

Most of all, she bridled at the blase attitude of family and friends, and even a health professional, toward "just a biopsy."

We need to realize and admit that a biopsy can

---

*LeeAn Lowe, "No Biopsy Is Routine," *Cosmopolitan*, October 1985, p. 42.

arouse strong feelings in us, and that the strange alchemy of our emotions can transform one too-painful feeling into another we can accept more easily. Thus, "If I have cancer, will I die?" becomes "I have to wait *how* long for this biopsy? This place isn't very well organized, it it?"

To face a biopsy is to face the possibility of serious disease—and one's own mortality. Doctor, nurse, spouse, friend can help, if we admit we need help. Getting accurate information and support, plus a chance to talk about our fears and uncertainties, gives us a chance to put our feelings into perspective, and to accept them and ourselves. It's the unacknowledged feelings that may seethe within.

On the other hand, accepted feelings are energy which we can use to recover quickly from a minor ordeal. The strengths we harness in ourselves to cope with this unknown are ones which can stand us in good stead all our lives.

When I underwent my first biopsy, many years ago, I visualized an *exhausting* number of scenarios beforehand. One moment I was convinced that all would be well, the procedure a snap, and the results benign. The next moment, I imagined my husband and small children gathered around my deathbed. In fact, my unbridled imagination suffered far more than the rest of me did!

I'll never love biopsies: They all bring some discomfort and apprehension. *But* the discomfort is short-lasting and, in most cases, the price—a brief period of heightened anxiety—is a reasonable one to pay for long-lasting relief from worry about a suspicious area. Even if the diagnosis is breast cancer, I think I'd rather know, and be able to take action after a biopsy, than to fret about what that peculiar breast lump might be.

By the second biopsy, I managed to eliminate *most* of the deathbed scenarios!

Reasonably
Happily Ever After

Once upon a time there lived a man and his wife, who said to each other every day of their lives, "Would that we had a child!" But for many years they had none.

At last though, as the years went by, the wife gave birth to a baby daughter so beautiful that the husband could not contain his joy. "She's just my little Princess," he said (which may or may not have a bearing on this story).

To celebrate the birth of their child, the man and his wife decided to hold a christening party for all the great aunts and wise women and old crones in the neighborhood. Alas, there were thirteen of them to invite—and the man and his wife had only twelve place settings of their china. So one of them was not invited.

The christening was celebrated with joy and merrymaking. When it came time for the gift giving, the most eccentric of the old women gave little Princess a sterling silver baby spoon and a dainty dress. But the others contented themselves with the conventional gifts: beauty, charm, impeccable fashion sense, a complexion neither too dry nor too oily—things like that.

As the twelfth guest prepared to bestow her gift, there was a great commotion. In stormed the uninvited thirteenth, yearning to revenge herself for the slight. Without greeting, she cried with a loud voice, "When she grows up, Princess will have lumpy, bumpy (and sometimes painful) breasts, and she will have to worry about breast cancer!" And without another word, she turned away and left.

Everyone was horrified at what had happened.

Then the twelfth guest came forward to give her gift. Though she could not undo the curse, she could soften it, so she said, "I bestow on Princess the gift of Common Sense, which will let her live comfortably with her lumpy, bumpy (and sometimes painful) breasts, and with her worry about breast cancer!"

Desiring to save their daughter from her fate, the man and his wife decided that no one would ever mention the word "breast" in their king. . .er, house.

Princess grew up, adorned with all the gifts of the great aunts and wise women and old crones. She was beautiful and charming, and had both an impeccable fashion sense and a complexion that was neither too dry nor too oily.

But it happened one day that Princess, now a young woman, read an article about breast cancer in a magazine. For the first time she encountered "the 7 warning signs of cancer" and "1 in every 10 women will get breast cancer." Soon afterwards, as she was showering one day, she happened to feel her soapy breasts. There was SOMETHING there—lumpy and bumpy (and sometimes painful)!

Poor Princess fell into a daze, and went about her activities as if she were sleepwalking.

"Mommy, Mommy! You're telling the story all wrong!"
"Hush, my darling, and listen. . ."

Now there was a gallant young man in the neighborhood—a real prince of a fellow—but unfortunately he had been called out of town at this time.

So the days and weeks went by, and the dazed Princess ate little and slept too much. Since her parents had never mentioned breasts to her, she had never learned what to do or where to turn.

But one day the sleepy Princess awakened and said to herself, "This is absolutely ridiculous. Get hold of yourself, my girl. I bet that if I looked around, I could find some information and some help. Maybe— just maybe—this isn't as bad as I think it is."

And thus did Common Sense come to the rescue!

"I'll find a doctor with whom I feel comfortable," said Princess. "I want someone who can, and will, answer my questions." And so Princess found a competent and compassionate doctor.

The doctor examined her breasts carefully, and told Princess that her breasts were lumpy and bumpy (and sometimes painful) because they were doing what they were supposed to be doing, with great enthusiasm. There was no sign of breast cancer.

Then the doctor and a nurse practitioner taught her how to examine her breasts carefully each month. They showed her the different structures and kinds of tissue in her breasts. They explained how she could use her eyes to see, her fingers to palpate—and her brain to perceive any changes.

And because she had Common Sense, Princess listened and practiced BSE faithfully, just as she brushed her teeth after meals. Princess knew that with her lumpy, bumpy (and sometimes painful) breasts, she needed to become very well acquainted with what was normal for her, so that she could spot any change quickly.

The doctor told Princess that she was still too young for a mammogram, but that mammography would become a useful tool for her when she became older.

Together, the doctor and Princess reviewed her risk factors for breast cancer, and set up a follow-up schedule which made them both content: how often she would see the doctor, when she would perform BSE, when she would start having mammograms. They also talked about pain relief, although Princess had already discovered that reassurance was one of the best painkillers available.

The commonsensical Princess realized that no one knows for sure how to *prevent* breast cancer, although diet may be a factor.

"I'll watch my diet, but I'm also putting my money on early *detection*," thought Princess. "If, by any chance, I ever develop breast cancer, I'm making sure it will be detected and diagnosed at an early stage—when it's curable.

"That doesn't mean that I'm never going to worry about my breasts. But it does mean that I feel in control of the situation.

"Yippee!"

And so Princess lived quite happily ever after, full of beauty, charm, and common sense (not to mention an impeccable fashion sense, and a complexion neither too dry nor too oily).

"The Prince, Mommy! What about the Prince?"

"Another night, my dear one. It's time for sleep now."

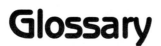

Glossary

acinus (alveolus) In the breast, one of the tiny sacs lined with gland cells which extract ingredients from nearby blood vessels and recombine them to produce milk. (plural: acini)

adenofibroma See **fibroadenoma**.

adenoma See **fibroadenoma**.

adenosis A benign breast change marked by an increase in the proportion of glandular (adeno-) tissue to the other kinds of tissue in the breast. This change is not associated with an increased risk of breast cancer.

> **sclerosing adenosis** A common form of adenosis which occurs in two phases: 1) a solid benign breast lump develops; 2) sclerosis (hardening) replaces the cells of the breast lump. If the areas of sclerosis calcify, they may lead to misleading findings on a mammogram.

alveolus See **acinus**. (plural: alveoli)

ampulla (sinus) In the breast, one of the small reservoirs for milk, located with one end under the areola. Milk drains into the ampulla from the duct of the breast, and is released from there through the nipple during breastfeeding. (plural: ampullae)

apocrine metaplasia A benign breast change in which the cells lining the breast ducts, normally shaped like cubes, become longer and shaped like columns. This change is not associated with an increased risk of breast cancer.

architecture of the breast The arrangement of the structures within the breast, including the tiny fibrous strands. Changes or distortions in the architecture can occur with benign or cancerous conditions and can sometimes be detected on a mammogram before there are any other indications of a problem.

areola   The pigmented (darker) area of the breast, roughly circular, around the base of the nipple. (plural: areolae or areolas)

aspiration   See **needle aspiration.**

atypia   The condition of having abnormal cells, different in appearance, internal organization, or behavior. Breast atypia is linked with an increased risk of breast cancer.

axilla   armpit area, which contains lymph nodes and channels, blood vessels, muscles, and fat. (plural: axillae)

benign   Not cancerous. A few kinds of benign breast changes are linked with an increased risk of breast cancer.

benign breast changes   (benign breast conditions, disorders, problems) An umbrella term for any alteration in the breast which is not cancerous.

biopsy   The surgical removal and microscopic examination of a piece of tissue to diagnose a problem.

> **conventional surgical biopsy**   Removal of a palpable lump or thickening by the surgeon.
>
> **excisional biopsy**   A biopsy which removes (excises) all of the questionable tissue.
>
> **incisional biopsy**   A procedure in which the surgeon cuts into (incises) a suspicious area and removes a small sample.
>
> **needle localization biopsy**   A special biopsy technique used when the breast abnormality cannot be felt with the fingers and appears only on mammography. Before biopsy, the radiologist marks the suspicious area with needle(s) and often dye. The surgeon then locates and removes the marked area of tissue, and the biopsy specimen is X-rayed to be sure all the suspicious area has been removed.

breast carcinoma in situ   (in situ breast carcinoma, non-invasive breast carcinoma, noninfiltrating breast carcinoma) A breast change in which highly atypical cells are localized; that is, they may press against adjoining breast tissue but they have not penetrated (invaded) it nor spread (metastasized) beyond the breast. Doctors differ about whether this condition marks the last stage of benign change or the first stage of breast cancer; it is associated with an increased risk of later invasive breast cancer.

duct carcinoma in situ   (DCIS, noninvasive duct carcinoma) A form of breast carcinoma in situ confined to the breast ducts which often reveals itself with tiny specks (microcalcifications) on a mammogram. The larger the area of DCIS, the greater the risk of invasive breast cancer.

lobular carcinoma in situ   (LCIS, lobular neoplasia) A form of breast carcinoma in situ characterized by multiple areas of highly atypical cells, often in both breasts. Occurs in the terminal ducts of the breast lobules. Extent of the situ areas is not related to the risk of invasive breast cancer.

Paget's disease of the nipple   A form of breast carcinoma in situ which often shows itself with an eczema-like rash of the nipple.

breast self-examination (BSE) Inspection and palpation of her breasts by the woman herself.

BSE   See **breast self-examination**.

calcifications   See **microcalcifications**.

chronic cystic mastitis   See **fibrocystic breast condition**.

colostrum   The thin, yellowish milk secreted by the breasts of the mother right before and right after the birth of her baby. It is especially suited to the needs of the newborn.

compressor   A device used during mammography to flatten the breast for more accurate X-rays.

computed tomography   (Computerized tomography, CT) A technique for imaging a body part using X-rays, special detectors, and computer equipment; used occasionally for breast imaging.

Cooper's ligaments   Flexible bands of fibrous tissue which pass from the chest muscle between the lobes of the breast and attach to the skin, giving the breast shape and support.

cyst   A fluid-filled lump in the breast, ordinarily benign.

macrocyst   A cyst large enough to feel with the fingers, which is drained during needle aspiration.

microcyst   A cyst too small to feel with the fingers.

cystosarcoma phylloides   See **fibroadenoma**.

cytology   The study of cells. In the cytology laboratory cells from the body are examined under a microscope for the presence of cancer.

DCIS   Duct carcinoma in situ. See **breast carcinoma in situ.**

density of breast tissue   A measure of the characteristic of some breast tissue which makes it more difficult to visualize in mammograms, caused by normal working breast tissue in young women, individual variations in breast structures, and some benign breast changes.

diaphanography   (transillumination) A technique for imaging the breast by directing infrared light through the breast, photographing the transmitted light with special film, and interpreting the film.

dimpling   See **retraction.**

dominant lump   In breast examination, a nodule that stands out from the surrounding breast tissue, three-dimensional and different from neighboring areas.

duct   A channel for transporting milk in the breast.

duct carcinoma in situ   See **breast carcinoma in situ.**

duct ectasia   A benign breast change in which large or small ducts in the breast become dilated and retain secretions, often leading to nipple discharge, and sometimes a lump in the nipple/areola area and/or nipple retraction. This change is not associated with an increased risk of breast cancer.

duct x-ray   A technique used occasionally for imaging the nipple and areola area ducts by injecting into a pore of the nipple a small amount of fluid visible on x-ray and then obtaining a mammogram.

estrogen   A female hormone which every month before menopause readies the breast for possible milk production and transport by multiplying and enlarging breast cells.

excisional biopsy   See **biopsy.**

fat necrosis   (traumatic fat necrosis) A benign breast change in which the breast responds to trauma (including surgical biopsy sometimes) with a firm, irregular mass, often years after the event. This breast change is not associated with an increased risk of breast cancer.

fibroadenoma   (adenoma, adenofibroma, fibroma) A benign breast condition common in young adult women in which the breast develops a solid lump, either firm or soft, but usually movable in the breast. The lump is named according to the proportions of gland (adeno-) and fibrous (fibro-) tissue present. This breast change is not associated with an increased risk of breast cancer.

cystosarcoma phylloides   A variation of a fibroadenoma, often very large and, on rare occasions, cancerous.

fibroadenosis   See **fibrocystic breast condition**.

fibrocystic breast condition   (fibrocystic breast disease or changes, chronic cystic mastitis, fibroadenosis, mastodynia, mammary dysplasia, benign breast changes) A term used to mean changes in the fibrous tissue in the breast with the formation of cysts or, more broadly, for any benign breast change. Common symptoms are general lumpiness in the breasts, cystic lumps, and tenderness.

fibroma   See **fibroadenoma**.

frozen section   A technique by which a tissue specimen from biopsy is quick-frozen, cut into thin slices, stained, and examined microscopically by a pathologist for immediate report to the surgeon. This report, often available while the woman is still in the operating room, is preliminary but about 98% accurate.

hyperplasia   An increase in the number of cells beyond the normal range. Small increases in the number of cells lining the breast ducts are not associated with an increased risk of cancer, but a greater degree of hyperplasia is associated with a slightly increased risk of breast cancer.

incisional biopsy   See **biopsy**.

in situ breast carcinoma   See **breast carcinoma in situ**.

inspection   The part of breast examination in which the breasts are examined visually.

invasive breast cancer   Disease in which breast cancer cells have penetrated (invaded) surrounding breast tissue.

inverted nipple   A condition in which the nipple, instead of protruding, is "inside out," tucked into the areola. If present since puberty, this is a normal variation; if it represents a change, and occurs in one breast, it may be a sign of either benign or cancerous breast conditions.

lactation   The process of producing milk and breastfeeding a child.

lactiferous   Milk-carrying, as applied to ducts and related structures in the breast.

LCIS   Locular carcinoma in situ. See **breast carcinoma in situ**.

lesion   A general term for a change in tissue structure or function due to injury or other processes. Most lesions are benign.

lipoma   A benign soft lump composed of fatty tissue. This change is not associated with an increased risk of breast cancer.

lobe   A portion of the breast which contains a complete unit for producing, transporting, and delivering milk. It consists of several acini and ducts, an ampulla, and a duct opening on the nipple. Each breast contains several lobes.

lobular carcinoma in situ   See **breast carcinoma in situ**.

lobular neoplasia   See **breast carcinoma in situ**.

lobule   A subdivision of a breast lobe.

lumpectomy   Removal of a lump and a small amount of surrounding breast tissue. Currently used as an option for some small breast cancers.

lymph node   A bean-shaped filter along the course of a lymph vessel through which tissue fluid normally drains. The node traps harmful organisms so that they don't enter the body's circulatory system. Breast examination includes a check of the lymph nodes in the armpit area for any swelling.

macrocyst   See **cyst**.

magnetic resonance imaging   (MRI—formerly called nuclear magnetic resonance, or NMR) An imaging technique which uses an interaction of magnetism and radiowaves to picture the interior of the breast.

magnification views   In mammography, a technique for producing an enlarged picture of a small area of suspicious breast tissue, providing greater detail for the radiologist who interprets the film.

mammary dysplasia   Literally, poorly structured tissue in the breast. For common use, see **fibrocystic breast condition**.

mammography   X-ray of the breast which often detects breast changes (including duct carcinoma in situ and invasive breast cancer) before they can be felt with the fingers. Mammography produces a black-and-white film mammogram.

xeromammography (Xeroradiography, pronounced "zero. . .") A variation on a mammogram which uses a recording techniqe developed by the Xerox Corporation to produce a blue-and-white X-ray picture on special paper.

mastectomy Surgical removal of all or part of the breast and sometimes adjoining structures, usually done for breast cancer.

    subcutaneous mastectomy Surgical removal of most of the breast tissue, which is replaced with a silicone gel implant. This procedure is sometimes done for a woman at high risk of breast cancer as a **prophylactic** (preventive) measure.

mastitis Inflammation of the breast. Commonly an acute benign condition, an infection which often occurs in women who are breastfeeding and is treated with antibiotics. It occasionally becomes a chronic condition. Mastitis is not associated with an increased risk of breast cancer.

    chronic cystic mastitis See **fibrocystic breast condition**.

methylxanthine A chemical substance found in caffeine. Some studies have found a connection between methylxanthines and breast lumpiness and/or pain, although other studies question the link.

microcalcifications (calcifications) Tiny white specks of calcium salts which can sometimes be seen on mammograms. In clusters, they can be the only sign of duct carcinoma in situ or early invasive cancer, or can be associated with benign breast changes.

microcyst See **cyst**.

monoclonal antibodies Laboratory-produced copies (clones) of cancer-fighting antibodies used in an experimental X-ray technique for detection of recurrent cancer.

Montgomery's tubercles Visible pores or tiny lumps on the areola, openings for the oil glands which lubricate the nipple and areola during breastfeeding.

needle aspiration (aspiration) A diagnostic technique in which a thin hypodermic needle is inserted into a lump which may be fluid-filled, and any fluid is withdrawn into the syringe. If the lump is a cyst, it collapses. Any suspicious fluid can be sent to the cytology laboratory for examination. Sometimes a special needle or a different technique is used to withdraw a tiny piece of tissue or several cells from a solid lump.

needle localization biopsy See **biopsy**.

nipple discharge Fluid which comes out of the nipple, either spontaneously or when the nipple area is squeezed. Nipple discharge (other than milk in a lactating woman) often results from benign breast changes or minor hormonal irregularities, but needs to be checked by a health professional.

nodularity General lumpiness.

nodule A lump.

noninfiltrating breast carcinoma See **breast carcinoma in situ**.

noninvasive breast carcinoma See **breast carcinoma in situ**.

non-proliferative breast changes Benign breast changes in which there is no cell multiplication beyond the limits of normal. These changes, such as fibroadenoma and cysts, are not associated with an increased risk of breast cancer.

Paget's disease of the nipple See **breast carcinoma in situ**.

palpation Generally, examination by touch. The part of breast examination during which the breast tissue and structures are felt with the fingers.

papilloma A benign finger-like growth in a breast duct.

parenchyma The "working" tissue of the breast, including the structures which produce, transport, and store milk.

permanent section The technique for producing definitive slides from biopsied tissue for the pathologist to interpret. The procedure takes about 24 hours and includes fixing the tissue in formaldehyde, processing it in various chemicals, slicing it very thin, and staining it. The slides produced are detailed and clear, and are examined by the pathologist for the final report.

progesterone A female hormone which puts the breast cells to work practicing or actually secreting milk in the premenopausal woman.

prolactin A female hormone which stimulates the development of the breasts and later is essential for starting and continuing milk production.

proliferative breast changes with atypia   Breast changes in which the cells multiply beyond the limits of normal and in which some cells are abnormal in appearance and/ or organization. This change is associated with a significantly increased risk of breast cancer; the more abnormal the cells, the greater the cancer risk.

proliferative breast changes without atypia   Breast changes in which the cells multiply beyond the limits of normal without apparent abnormal cells. This change is associated with a slightly increased risk of breast cancer.

prophylactic mastectomy   See **mastectomy**.

retraction   (dimpling) A visual change in either the breast contour or the nipple, often caused by an alteration in the tension of a Cooper's ligament on the skin or nipple. The skin develops a dip, dimple, or hollow, seen best when the chest muscles are contracted, or the nipple changes its axis or protrusion. Benign changes can cause retraction, but a cancerous tumor, attaching to the ligament, can cause this change even before there's a lump to feel.

sclerosing adenosis   See **adenosis**.

specimen radiography   The technique for examining a biopsy specimen by X-ray. When a biopsy has been performed because of abnormalities seen on mammogram, this X-ray confirms that all the questionable area has been removed.

stellate   Star-shaped, referring to an unusual arrangement of breast fibers sometimes seen on mammography, suspicious for breast cancer although it occurs with benign conditions also.

stroma   The components of breast tissue which give it shape and support (fat and fibrous tissue) but do not participate in milk production and transport.

subcutaneous mastectomy   See **mastectomy**.

thermography   A breast imaging technique which measures body heat at the skin level to identify hot spots due to inflammation or cancer.

transillumination   See **diaphanography**.

traumatic fat necrosis   See **fat necrosis**.

ultrasound   A breast imaging technique in which high-frequency sound waves are painlessly projected into the breast and the pattern of echoes is interpreted.

xeromammography   See **mammography**.

Index

Glossary page numbers appear in bold-faced type.

150

"wide needle" aspiration 121–2

Xeromammography 106, **143**. See also mammography
Xeroradiography, see xeromammography